D1098936

Pocket
Emergency
Paediatric
Care

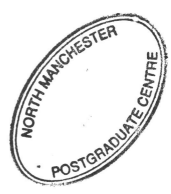

Pocket
Emergency
Paediatric
Care

A practical guide to the diagnosis and management of
paediatric emergencies in hospitals and other healthcare
facilities worldwide

Shafique Ahmad
and
David Southall
Child Advocacy International,
Newcastle Under Lyme, UK
and
Child Advocacy International,
Registered Charity 1071486

© BMJ Books 2003
BMJ Books is an imprint of the BMJ Publishing Group

First published in 2003
Second impression 2004
by BMJ Books, BMA House, Tavistock Square,
London WC1H 9JR

www.bmjbooks.com

British Library Cataloguing in Publication Data

A catalogue record for this book is available from the British Library

ISBN 0 7279 1701 3

Cover image © image100 Ltd
Cover design by Egelnick and Webb

Typeset by SIVA Math Setters, Chennai, India
Printed and bound in Spain by GraphyCems, Navarra

Contents

Preface   vii
Acknowledgements   ix
UNCRC standards   xi

Section 1: Life-threatening emergencies   1
Essential knowledge   3
Triage   7
Resuscitation at birth   9
Paediatric life support   11
Recognition of the sick child   16
The shocked child   22
The unconscious child   26
Allergic reactions and anaphylactic shock   35
Status epilepticus   37
Poisoning   39

Section 2: Neonatal emergencies   47
Fluid and electrolyte balance in the ill neonate   49
Hypoglycaemia in the neonate   51
Hypoglycaemia in the ill neonate   52
Jaundice in the ill neonate   54
Respiratory problems in the neonate   57
Neonatal infections   59
Neonatal seizures   62
Neonatal hypoxic ischaemic encephalopathy (HIE)   64

Section 3: Specific emergencies   65
Respiratory and cardiovascular   67
Gastrointestinal/liver/renal   75
Neurological   98

Endocrine and metabolic   104
Infectious diseases   111
Environmental emergencies   127
Trauma and surgical emergencies   136

Section 4: Procedures and equipment   149

Section 5: Appendices   169

Index   195

Preface

This book is designed to fit into a handbag or shirt pocket. It contains material which is usually required in a hurry when treating a critically ill or injured infant or child. In addition to information relevant to emergency care, there are what we hope will be useful pages of data on subjects which without a photographic memory would normally require reference to a paediatric text book. Examples include a weight for height chart, normal values for common biochemical tests, normal developmental profiles and normal ECG measurements.

Finally, this book is meant to be used by paediatricians and nurses working in hospitals all over the world. The authors recognise that in many poorly resourced States the standards required to achieve the levels of critical care outlined here will not always be practical. However, our view is that all children are entitled to minimum standards of care, as outlined in the United Nations Convention on the Rights of the Child (see page xi) and that advocacy to achieve these might be aided by this publication and by the actions of the healthcare workers who use it.

Acknowledgements

The contents of this pocket book originate from a recent publication entitled *International Child Health Care: a practical manual for hospitals worldwide*, published by BMJ Books and Child Advocacy International. Emergency and critical care components which are chapters in the latter book, have been extracted and summarised. We are therefore particularly grateful to the original editors of the manual – Dr B Coulter, Dr C Ronald, Dr S Nicholson and Dr S Parke.

We also thank the following chapter authors:

Dr Alastair Baker, Professor Zulfiqar Bhutta, Dr Luz Marina Lozano Chavarria, Andrew Clarke, Dr Nick Coleman, Dr Ed Cooper, Dr Malcolm Coulthard, Dr Ariel Dhawan, Dr Christopher Duke, Professor Michael Golden, Professor Nick Guerina, Dr Devendra Kurnar Gupta, Dr James Hagadorn, Dr Ismeta Kalkan, Dr Leela Kapila, Dr Anupam Lall, Dr David Lalloo, Professor Michael Levin, Dr Mary Limebury, Dr Steve Mannion, Dr Waghi El Masri, Professor Elizabeth Molyneux, Dr Sarah Morley, Dr Robert Moy, Dr Charles Newton, Dr Peter Oakley, Dr Bernhards Ogutu, Dr Deb Pal, Dr Silvia Patrizi, Dr Barbara Phillips, Dr Shakeel Qureshi, Dr Anthony Roberts, Dr Joan Robson, Dr Oliver Ross, Dr Martin Samuels, Dr Manoj Shenoy, Dr Alan Smyth, Professor Taunton Southwood, Dr Peter Sullivan, Professor R Theakston, Dr Sirijitt Vasanawathana, Dr Jerry Wales, Dr Mary Warrell, Dr Anthony Williams, Dr Gareth Tudor Williams, Dr Bridget Wills.

We are also grateful to the editors of the manual of *Advanced Paediatric Life Support* (also published by BMJ Books), which provided much of the information on emergencies and critical care.

Finally we thank Dr P McCormick for contributions to the malaria section, Dr Marion Schmidt for her help with the neonatal section, and Dr M Samuels for his assistance with proofreading this book.

UNCRC standards

Health care providers, organisations and individuals, share a responsibility to advocate for children and to reduce their fear, anxiety and suffering by ensuring that:

1. They admit and keep a child in an inpatient health facility only when this is in the child's and family's best interests*.
2. They provide the highest attainable (best possible) appropriate* level of care, evidence-based where possible.
3. The environment is secure, safe and clean.
4. They provide separate age and developmental appropriate care in partnership* with parents in child and family friendly surroundings.
5. They keep children and their parents/carers consistently and fully informed and involved in all decisions affecting care.
6. They give children equal access to health services and treat them as individuals without discrimination, with their own cultural, age and developmental appropriate rights to privacy, dignity, respect and confidentiality.
7. They assess and control children's physical and psychological pain and discomfort.
8. They provide appropriate* critical and emergency care for children that are severely ill, undergoing surgery, or have been given systemic analgesia and/or sedation.
9. Children are able to play and learn.
10. They recognise, protect and support abused children.
11. They monitor and promote health.
12. They support breastfeeding and the optimal nourishment of children.

*For definitions of the terminology used, please refer to the CFHI definitions – www.childfriendlyhealthcare.org

A STANDARD = a professionally agreed level of performance, appropriate to the population addressed, which is observable, achievable, measurable and desirable

Each of the above Standards is supported by a number of key components (supporting criteria). These Standards and their supporting criteria attempt to encompass all aspects of health care for children.

Life-threatening emergencies

Essential knowledge

Weight: (1 kg = 2·2 lb)

Infant: 0–1 years = 3–10 kg
5 months: double birth weight
12 months: treble birth weight
After 1 year: wt in kg = 2 (age + 4)
2 years: quadruple birth weight.

Airway and breathing (endotracheal intubation) – under 25 kg = uncuffed

Full term infant = 3·0–3·5 mm ID
Infant < 1 year = 4·0–4·5 mm ID
Child > 1 year = age/4 + 4 ID.
Length of tube = $\left[\dfrac{\text{Age}}{2}\right]$ + 12 cm for oral tube
+ 14 cm for nasal tube

Circulation (dehydration treatment: deficit in ml = % dehydration × weight in kg × 10)

Blood pressure systolic = 80 + (age year × 2) **Cuff must be
two-thirds size of upper arm and the largest that will fit**
Capillary refill = 2 seconds or less after 5 seconds pressure
(sternum)
Drip rates for clear fluids: (standard giving set)
20 drops = 1 ml
ml/h divided by 3 = drops/min
Minimum urine output: > 1 ml/kg/h in children, > 2 ml/kg/h
in infants
Insensible losses: 300 ml/m^2/24 h or

12 ml/kg/24 h if > 1 year
15 ml/kg/24 h if an infant
24 ml/kg/24 h if preterm
increased if in hot climate by around 50%
increased if fever by 50%

Fluid management

Blood volume is 100 ml/kg at birth falling to 80 ml/kg at
1 year. Total body water varies from 800 ml/kg in the neonate
to 600 ml/kg at one year and thereafter. Of this about two
thirds (400 ml/kg) is intracellular. Clinically, dehydration is
not detectable until >5% (50 ml/kg).

Fluid requirements:

1. Replace *insensible losses* through sweat, respiration,
    gastrointestinal loss etc.
2. Replace of *essential urine output*, the minimal urine output
    to allow excretion of the products of metabolism etc.
3. Extra fluid to maintain a *modest state of diuresis*.
4. Fluid to replace *abnormal losses* such as blood loss,
    severe diarrhoea, diabetic polyuria losses etc.

Normal fluid requirements

Body weight	Fluid requirement per day	Fluid requirement per hour
First 10 kg	100 ml/kg	4 ml/kg
Second 10 kg	50 ml/kg	2 ml/kg
Subsequent kg	20 ml/kg	1 ml/kg

Examples: 6 kg infant would require 600 ml per day
14 kg child would require 1000 + 200 = 1200 ml per day
25 kg child would require 1000 + 500 + 100 = 1600 ml per day.

Electrolyte contents of body fluids

Fluid	Na (mmol/1)	K (mmol/l)	Cl (mmol/l)	HCO3 (mmol/l)
Plasma	135–141	3·5–5·5	100–105	24–28
Gastric	20–80	5–20	100–150	0
Intestinal	100–140	5–15	90–130	15–65
Diarrhoea	7–96	34–150	17–164	0–75
Sweat	<40	6–15	<40	0–10

Normal water, electrolyte, energy and protein requirements (provided excessive loss is not present)

Body weight	Water (ml/kg/day)	Sodium (mmol/kg/day)	Potassium (mmol/kg/day)	Energy (kcal/day)	Protein (g/day)
First 10 kg	100	2–4	1·5–2·5	110	3·00
Second 10 kg	50	1–2	0·5–1·5	75	1·50
Subsequent kg	20	0·5–1·0	0·2–0·7	30	0·75

Essential drug doses

Aminophylline: IV loading dose 5 mg/kg over 20 minutes (max = 250 mg) then 1 mg/kg/h by IV infusion

Benzyl penicillin: 50 mg/kg IV 4–6 hourly

Cefotaxime: IV 50 mg/kg 6 hourly

Diazepam IV or IO 100–250 micrograms/kg or rectal 500 micrograms/kg (max = 10 mg)

Lorazepam IV or IO 50–100 micrograms/kg

Paraldehyde rectal or IM 0·4 ml/kg (max 10 ml rectal, 5 ml IM at one site)

Epinephrine (adrenaline): 10 micrograms/kg (0·1 ml/kg 1 in 10 000 or 0·01 ml/kg of 1 in 1000)

Epinephrine: 1 in 1000 = 1 mg/ml: 1 in 10 000 = 100 micrograms/ml

Fluid resuscitation: 20 ml/kg 0·9% saline or colloid or blood (10 ml/kg in neonate)

Frusemide: 1 mg/kg IV

Glucose: 5 ml/kg of 10% IV (0.5 g/kg)

Mannitol: 250–500 mg/kg IV over 20 minutes

Morphine: IV 100 micrograms/kg over 5 minutes (50–100 micrograms/kg in the neonate)

Salbutamol: 100–1000 micrograms inhaler (1–10 sprays) or nebuliser (dose 2·5 mg < 5 years and 5 mg > 5 years)

Salbutamol: IV loading dose = 4–6 micrograms/kg over 15 minutes monitor ECG and ensure K^+ normal

Sodium bicarbonate: 1 mmol/kg (= 2 ml/kg of 4·2%).

Disability

Assessment of neurological function (AVPU) (see page 29 for modified Glasgow Coma Scale)

A = alert, V = responds to voice, P = responds to pain, U = unresponsive.

Pupillary size and reaction, posture, muscle tone, presence of convulsive movements.

Normal values for paediatric vital signs in patients who are not crying

Age	Heart rate	Systolic blood pressure	Respiratory rate
< 1 year	120–140	70–90	30–40
2–5 years	100–120	80–90	20–30
5–12 years	80–100	90–110	15–20

Triage

Seeing the sickest first: triage

Triage is an important component of critical care, especially in resource poor settings.

Cards given to parents containing their triage classification and timing of assessment can be useful. Different colours and time codes can be an easy way of efficiently scoring the patients.

Urgent signs from one such triage system are illustrated below.

Emergency signs, assessment and treatment (adapted from WHO)

Area of assessment	Clinical signs	Result	Treatment If any sign positive or coma or convulsing: give treatment(s), call for help, draw emergency bloods (glucose, malaria smear, Hb, electrolytes) then assess response to initial treatment
1. Assess airway and breathing	• Obstructed breathing or • Central cyanosis or • Severe respiratory distress	ANY SIGN POSITIVE	• Manage airway • Give oxygen • Make sure child is warm
2. Assess circulation →	Shock • Capillary refill > 2 s after 5 s pressure on sternum • Cold/pale/sweating • Weak and fast pulse • Bradycardia? (Listen with stethoscope)	ANY SIGN POSITIVE Check for severe malnutrition	• Stop any bleeding • Give oxygen • Make sure child is warm IF NO SEVERE MALNUTRITION: • Insert IV line and give 10–20 ml/kg 0·9% saline or colloid as rapidly as possible. If not able to insert peripheral IV line, insert external jugular,

Continued

Area of assessment	Clinical signs	Result	Treatment If any sign positive or coma or convulsing: give treatment(s), call for help, draw emergency bloods (glucose, malaria smear, Hb, electrolytes) then assess response to initial treatment
			femoral venous, long saphenous cut-down or intraosseous line IF SEVERE MALNUTRITION: • Give IV glucose 5 ml/kg 10% • Proceed to full assessment and treatment (see page 79)
3. Assess neurological state →	• Agitated or depressed consciousness • Coma or • Convulsing (now)	IF COMA OR CONVULSING Check for head/neck trauma before treating child— stabilise neck if cervical spine injury possible (see page 138)	• Manage airway • Position child • Give O_2 • If convulsing, give diazepam rectally (500 micrograms/kg) 2·5 mg if < 1year, 5 mg if 1–3 years and 10 mg > 3 years • If no response give IV lorazepam 100 micrograms/kg or IV diazepam 250 micrograms/kg • Give IV glucose 5 ml/kg 10% or 2 ml/kg of 25% • Make sure child is warm

Resuscitation at birth

Initial assessment: note time (start clock)

- Colour (pink, blue, white)
- Tone
- Breathing (?apnoea)
- Heart rate (with stethoscope).

If not breathing CONTROL AIRWAY

- Neutral position of neck/head
- Towel under shoulders
- SUPPORT BREATHING
- 5 breaths of 2–3 seconds duration (blow off valve set at 30–45 cmH$_2$O)
- CONFIRM RESPONSE
- Visible chest movement or HR increases and improvement in colour.

If no response

- Check head position, try jaw thrust
- Repeat 5 breaths.

If no response

- Inspect airway, observed suction (ideally with laryngoscope)
- Insert oropharyngeal airway
- Consider intubation
- Repeat 5 breaths.

If chest expands: check heart rate.

If HR < 60 and not increasing give chest compressions (one-third depth)

- Confirm chest expansion
- 3 chest compressions to one inflation.

Reassess: if no response consider venous access and drugs.

Drugs: IV, UVC

Epinephrine (adrenaline): 10 micrograms/kg (0·1 ml/kg 1 in
    10 000 or 0·01 ml/kg 1 in 1000)

Epinephrine: 1 in 1000 = 1 mg/ml; 1 in 10 000 = 100
    micrograms/ml

Glucose: 5 ml/kg of 10%

Sodium bicarbonate: 1 mmol/kg (2 ml/kg of 4·2%)

Fluid resuscitation: 10 ml/kg 0·9% saline or colloid or blood.

Only epinephrine: 100 micrograms/kg, can be given via
endotracheal tube (that is 1 ml/kg of 1 in 10 000).

Paediatric life support

Shout for help

Approach with care (safety for yourself)

Free from danger (safety for your patient)

Evaluate ABC.

Check responsiveness – "Are you all right?"

Airway opening (neutral position for infant: sniffing for
child = neck extended, nasal orifices to vertical).

LOOK, LISTEN, FEEL – for respiration for 10 seconds.
Give 2–5 rescue breaths if breathing absent or ineffective.

Check pulse – brachial in infant, carotid in child and/or heart
rate with stethoscope for 10 seconds. Look for "signs of
life", for example movement, breathing. Check time (start
clock).

First priority – establish airway and ventilation

Open airway – head tilt (neutral – infant towel under
shoulders; sniffing – child), chin lift and jaw thrust (beware
of cervical spine injury: if suspected use jaw thrust without
head tilt).

Only do suction if airway blocked or filled with blood or
vomit – thin secretions not important: use Yankauer suction
catheter. Provide 5 initial breaths with self-inflating bag with
reservoir and 100% oxygen.

In absence of severe upper airway obstruction, adequate
ventilation should be obtained.

After 2–5 rescue breaths, do pulse check and support
circulation if required (i.e. don't stick to A and B for 5
minutes and forget pulse).

If unable to inflate chest – check airway position.

Still unable to inflate chest – try oro-pharyngeal airway.

Still unable to inflate chest – **consider intubation**:

ET tube size in full-term newborn infant: 3–3·5 mm

ET tube size in child ± 0·5 = (age/4) + 4 mm.

ET tube size in infant < 1 year: 4–4·5 mm.

Depth of insertion: 3 × internal diameter = length at lips in centimetres, add 2 cm at nares.

Uncuffed tube under 25 kg.

Ensure tube is passed only 2–3 cm below vocal cords – the black line on the ET tube should *just* pass through the cords.

After intubation check that lung inflation is occurring and that chest wall expansion is adequate and equal. Chest movement is the most useful sign. Auscultate in axillae and over epigastrium. Ensure no air bubbling up from mouth or heard in neck with stethoscope. Ventilate approximately every 2 seconds. Don't forget mouth to mouth/mouth and nose, or mouth to mask if self-inflating bag unavailable.

CXR to check endotracheal tube position – if prolonged ventilation needed. Failure to ventilate effectively may be due to incorrectly placed tube (oesophagus or right main bronchus) or consider pneumothorax.

Second priority – establish cardiac output

Cardiac massage (ratio of compression to ventilation: 3 : 1 in neonates, 5 : 1 in infants and children): 5 : 2 in older children where both hands are needed for compressions.

Firm surface (board, floor, examination couch).

Infants: two fingers, one finger breadth below the internipple line or use thumbs with hands encircling the chest wall.

Small children (< 8 years): use one hand to depress the sternum, one finger breadth above xiphisternum.

Larger children (> 8 years): heels of both hands are used to depress the sternum two finger breadths above xiphisternum.

Compress by one-third of AP diameter of chest. Effective massage produces femoral pulses. Rate 100/min

Usual reason for ineffective massage is insufficient
compression. Tamponade is a rare cause.

Third priority – attach to ECG monitor, if available

Fourth priority – establish intravenous access

Peripheral, intraosseous, femoral/internal jugular, cut down
long saphenous.

Consider correctable factors:

Severe dehydration/shock: start 0·9% saline 20 ml/kg boluses
syringe in quickly.

Haemorrhage: start O rhesus negative blood 20 ml/kg initially
IV/IO.

Drug therapy

Epinephrine (adrenaline)

Give 10 micrograms/kg (0·01 ml/kg of 1 in 1000 solution) IV
or intraosseous (IO) and flush with 3–5 ml 0·9% saline or give
100 micrograms/kg(0·1 ml/kg of 1 in 1000 solution) via ET
tube. For subsequent doses multiply the IV/IO dose by 10
(i.e. 0·1 ml/kg of 1 in 1000) in cases where shock caused the
cardiac arrest.

Sodium bicarbonate

When pH < 7·0 or cardiac output compromised, use
1 mmol/kg (2 ml/kg of 4·2%). **Do not use intratracheal
route**. *Bicarbonate* must not be given in same IV line as
calcium. *Sodium bicarbonate* inactivates epinephrine and
dopamine, therefore flush line with 0·9% saline if these drugs
are subsequently given.

Protocol for cardiac asystole

Continuous and effective life support

Ventilate 100% oxygen
IV or IO access
Intubate

Epinephrine: 10 micrograms/kg (0·01 ml/kg of 1 in 1000 or
0·1 ml/kg of 1 in 10 000) IV or IO or 100 micrograms/kg down
ET tube.

Give 3 minutes of cardiopulmonary resuscitation cycles

Consider IV fluid bolus (20 ml/kg of 0·9% saline) and sodium
bicarbonate 1 mmol/kg = 2 ml/kg of 4·2% IV or IM (never
intratracheally)

Repeat epinephrine 10–100 micrograms/kg (0·1 ml/kg of 1 in 10000 or 1000) IV or IO
Repeat 3 minutes of cardiopulmonary resuscitation cycles

Repeat cycle of last two lines in box

Protocol for pulseless electrical activity (PEA)
(ECG looks normal or bradycardia but no palpable pulse)

Continuous and effective life support

Ventilate 100% oxygen
IV or IO access
Intubate

Epinephrine: 10 micrograms/kg (0·01 ml/kg of 1 in 1000 or
0·1 ml/kg of 1 in 10 000) IV or IO or 100 micrograms/kg
down ET tube.
Fluids: IV bolus of 20 ml/kg.

Consider: hypovolaemia, tension pneumothorax, cardiac tamponade, drug

overdose, electrolyte imbalance and treat appropriately

Repeat epinephrine 10—100 micrograms/kg (0·1 ml/kg of 1 in 10000 or 1000) IV or IO

Repeat 3 minutes of cardiopulmonary resuscitation cycles

Repeat cycle of last two items in box

Protocol for ventricular fibrillation and pulseless VT

DC shock 2 J/kg
DC shock 2 J/kg
DC shock 4 J/kg

Continuous and effective life support

Ventilate with 100% oxygen
IV or IO access

Epinephrine: 10 micrograms/kg (0·01 ml/kg of 1 in 1000 or
0·1 ml/kg of 1 in 10 000 IV or IO) or 100 micrograms/kg
down ET tube.

DC shock 4 J/kg

DC shock 4 J/kg

DC shock 4 J/kg

Consider sodium bicarbonate 1 mmol/kg = 2 ml/kg of 4·2% IV but

never intratracheally

Consider antiarrhythmic drugs (for example, amiodarone, lignocaine)

Repeat epinephrine 10—100 micrograms/kg (0·1 ml/kg of 1 in 10000 or 1000) IV or IO

1 minute of cardiopulmonary resuscitation cycles from drugs to shock

Consider hypothermia, drugs and electrolyte imbalance

Repeat cycle of last eight items in box

Recognition of the sick child

Early recognition and management of potential respiratory, circulatory, or central neurological failure will reduce mortality and secondary morbidity.

The sections below describe the signs used for rapid assessment of children as part of the primary assessment:

Airway
Breathing
Circulation
Disability.

Primary assessment of airway

Vocalisations, such as crying or talking, indicate ventilation and some degree of airway patency.

Assess patency by:

looking for chest and/or abdominal movement
listening for breath sounds
feeling for expired air.

Reassess after any airway opening manoeuvres

In addition, note other signs which may suggest upper airway obstruction:

the presence of stridor
evidence of suprasternal recession ("tug").

Primary assessment of breathing

Assess:
Effort of breathing

Beware exceptions (fatigue, poisoning, neuromuscular diseases)
Efficacy of breathing
Effects of respiratory failure.

Effort of breathing

- Respiratory rate:
    tachypnoea – from either lung or airway disease or
        metabolic acidosis
    bradypnoea – due to fatigue, raised intracranial
        pressure, or pre-terminal.
- Recession:
    intercostal, subcostal or sternal recession shows
        increased effort of breathing
    particularly seen in small infants with more compliant
        chest walls
    degree of recession indicates severity of respiratory
        difficulty
    in the child with exhaustion, chest movement and
        recession will decrease.
- Inspiratory or expiratory noises:
    stridor, usually inspiratory, indicates laryngeal or
        tracheal obstruction
    wheeze, predominantly expiratory, indicates lower
        airway obstruction
    volume of noise is not an indicator of severity.
- Grunting:
    seen in infants and children with stiff lungs to prevent
        airway collapse
    it is a sign of severe respiratory distress
    it may also occur in intracranial and intra-abdominal
        emergencies.
- Accessory muscle use:
    in infants, the use of the sternomastoid muscle creates
        "head bobbing" and is ineffectual
    flaring of nasal alae.

Exceptions

Increased effort of breathing DOES NOT occur in three
circumstances:

exhaustion

central respiratory depression, for example from raised
   intracranial pressure, poisoning, or encephalopathy

neuromuscular disease, for example spinal muscular atrophy,
   muscular dystrophy or poliomyelitis.

Efficacy of breathing

- Breath sounds on auscultation:
    reduced or absent
    bronchial.
- Symmetrical or asymmetrical chest expansion – (most
  important)/abdominal excursion.
- Pulse oximetry. Normal SaO_2 in an infant or child at sea
  level is 95–100%. In air, this gives a good indication of the
  efficacy of breathing. SaO_2 at altitude may be lower.

Effects of respiratory failure on other physiology

- Heart rate:
    increased by hypoxia, fever, or stress
    bradycardia is a pre-terminal sign.
- Skin colour:
    hypoxia first causes vasoconstriction and pallor (via
      catecholamine release)
    cyanosis is a late and pre-terminal sign
    some children with congenital heart disease may be
      permanently cyanosed and oxygen may have
      little effect.
- Mental status:
    hypoxic or hypercapnic child will be agitated first,
      subsequently drowsy and then unconscious
    pulse oximetry may be difficult to achieve in the agitated
      child due to movement artefact.

Primary assessment of the circulation

Assess:
Circulatory status
Effects of circulatory inadequacy on other organs
Cardiac failure.

Circulatory status

- Heart rate.
- Pulse volume:
    absent peripheral pulses or reduced central pulses
      indicate shock.
- Capillary refill:
    pressure on the centre of the sternum or a digit for
      5 seconds should be followed by return of the
      circulation in the skin within 2 seconds
    may be prolonged by shock or cold environmental
      temperatures
    neither a specific nor sensitive sign of shock
    should not be used alone as a guide to the response
      to treatment.
- Blood pressure:
    cuff should be more than two thirds of the length of the
      upper arm and the bladder more than 40% of the
      arm's circumference
    hypotension is a late and pre-terminal sign of circulatory
      failure
    expected systolic BP = 80 + (age in years × 2). (see
    Appendix, p 189)

Effects of circulatory inadequacy on other organs/physiology

- Respiratory system:
    tachypnoea and hyperventilation occurs with acidosis.
- Skin:
    pale or mottled skin colour indicates poor perfusion.

- Mental status:
    agitation, then drowsiness leading to unconsciousness.
- Urinary output:
    < 1 ml/kg/h (< 2 ml/kg/h in infants) indicates inadequate
    renal perfusion.

Features suggesting cardiac cause of circulatory inadequacy:
    cyanosis, not correcting with oxygen therapy
    tachycardia out of proportion to respiratory difficulty
    raised jugular venous pressure
    gallop rhythm/murmur
    enlarged liver
    absent femoral pulses.

Primary assessment of disability

Always assess and treat airway, breathing, and circulatory
problems before undertaking the neurological assessment.

Respiratory and circulatory failure will have central
neurological effects.

Central neurological conditions (for example, meningitis,
raised intracranial pressure, status epilepticus) will have both
respiratory and circulatory consequences.

Neurological function
Respiratory effects
Circulatory effects

Neurological function
Conscious level – **AVPU** (a painful central stimulus may be
applied by sternal pressure or by pulling frontal hair):

Alert
responsive to **V**oice
responsive to **P**ain
Unresponsive.

- Posture:

  hypotonia

  decorticate or decerebrate postures (may only be elicited by a painful stimulus).

  opisthotonus for meningism or upper airway obstruction

- Pupils:

  pupil size, reactivity and symmetry

  dilatation, unreactivity or inequality indicate serious brain disorders.

Respiratory effects

Raised intracranial pressure may induce:

Hyperventilation
Cheynes–Stokes breathing
Slow, sighing respiration
Apnoea.

Circulatory effects

Raised intracranial pressure may induce:

Systemic hypertension
Sinus bradycardia.

The shocked child

Key features from a focused history

- Diarrhoea, vomiting = **fluid loss** either externally (for example, gastroenteritis, especially infants) or into abdomen (for example, volvulus, intussuception, initial stage of gastroenteritis).
- Fever and/or purpuric rash = **septicaemia**.
- Urticaria, angioneurotic oedema, and allergen exposure = **anaphylaxis**.
- Cyanosis unresponsive to oxygen with heart failure in a baby < 4 weeks = **duct-dependent congenital heart disease**.
- Heart failure in an older infant or child = severe anaemia or **cardiomyopathy**.
- Sickle cell disease, recent diarrhoeal illness, and very low haemoglobin = **acute haemolysis**.
- An immediate history of major trauma points to **blood loss** and, more rarely, **tension pneumothorax, haemothorax, cardiac tamponade**, or **spinal cord transection**.
- Severe tachycardia and abnormal rhythm on ECG = **arrhythmia**.
- Polyuria, acidotic breathing, high blood glucose = **diabetes**.
- Possible ingestion = **poisoning**.

Specific examination of cardiovascular status

Heart rate

Tachycardia common. Bradycardia results from hypoxaemia and acidosis and is pre-terminal.

Pulse volume

Poor pulse volume peripherally or, more worryingly, centrally. In early septic shock sometimes a high output state with bounding pulses.

Capillary refill

Slow capillary refill (> 2 seconds) after blanching pressure for 5 seconds on skin of the sternum. Mottling, pallor, and peripheral cyanosis also indicate poor skin perfusion. Difficult to interpret in patients exposed to cold.

Blood pressure

Blood pressure difficult to measure and interpret especially in young infants. Normal systolic BP = 80 + (2 × age in years). Hypotension is a late and often sudden sign of decompensation.

Effects of circulatory inadequacy on other organs

Acidotic sighing respirations.
Agitation or depressed conscious level.
Urinary output decreased or absent. A minimum flow of
    1 ml/kg/h in children and 2 ml/kg/h in infants indicates
    adequate renal perfusion.
Muscle tone: usually hypotonic.

Treatment of shock

ABC.
Oxygen 100%, reservoir mask.
IV cannula of widest bore (femoral, antecubital, or cut down or IO).

Fluid resuscitation immediately – 20 ml/kg of crystalloid or colloid as fast as possible. Syringe into patient. **Do not use dextrose solutions.** Reassess and repeated boluses of 20 ml/kg if shock persists.

Note: very large volumes of fluid resuscitation may be required early, especially in meningococcal infection and Dengue haemorrhagic fever. Use either 0·9% sodium chloride or colloid such as 4·5% human albumin. Blood products such as packed cells, fresh frozen plasma, and platelets may be required.

- Patients who remain shocked after 40 ml/kg colloid/crystalloid will probably benefit from inotropic support, for example dopamine 10–20 micrograms/kg/min IV (ideally central vein) or epinephrine 0·05–2·0 microgram/kg/min.
- Shocked patients are at risk of pulmonary oedema as fluid therapy increases. Ideal therapy is mechanical ventilation with PEEP for patients receiving > 40 ml/kg fluids. If pulmonary oedema develops (for example, tachypnoea, hypoxia, cough and fine crackles, raised jugular venous pressure, and hepatomegaly) further fluid withheld until stable. Give inotropes.
- Full neurological and cardiovascular assessment with regular (at least hourly) assessment of: pupillary responses, conscious level, pulse, blood pressure, capillary refill time, respiratory rate and effort (pulse oximetry if available), and temperature.
- Regular (ideally 4 hourly initially) monitoring of electrolytes (sodium, potassium, calcium and magnesium, phosphate, urea and/or creatinine) and glucose and replacement of deficits. Blood gas. Severe metabolic acidosis (pH < 7·1), which does not respond to fluid therapy, and inotropes may require sodium bicarbonate correction. Regular blood gas monitoring essential for ventilated patients.
- Monitor FBC and coagulation regularly if initially abnormal. Replacement of red cells to maintain Hb around 12 g/dL. Platelets and coagulation factors (usually FFP and cryoprecipitate) replaced as required to prevent bleeding.
- Hydration usually IV but NG feeding if tolerated. Urine output monitored (by indwelling catheter if conscious level depressed). NG for gastric drainage if persistent vomiting or decreased conscious level.

- If purpuric rash or other signs of septicaemia (after blood culture) IV antibiotic such as cefotaxime 50–100 mg/kg.
- Fluids ideally warmed, *but do not delay if not possible. Mother can place fluid bag next to her skin under dress to warm it*.
- 5 ml/kg 10% glucose IV (especially young child or infant) – after blood glucose test if available.
- If bleeding or severe anaemia FBC, clotting, group and cross-match, give type-specific, non-cross-matched blood ABO and rhesus compatible (but has a higher incidence of transfusion reactions) (takes 15 minutes) if cannot wait 1 hour for full cross-match. In dire emergencies O rhesus negative uncross-matched.
- If shock present and secondary to tachyarrhythmia:

Identify rhythm, attach to ECG monitor, obtain 12 lead ECG if possible

SVT

High flow oxygen

Attempt vagal manoeuvres, establish IV/IO access

No effect then use adenosine 50 micrograms/kg, then 100 micrograms/kg, then 250 micrograms/kg. Give as rapid boluses with rapid saline flush.

If unsuccessful three synchronous electrical shocks at 0·5, 1·0 and 2 J/kg (following rapid sequence induction of anaesthesia if conscious)

(VT)

If arrythmia is broad complex, pulse is present but in shock use synchronous shocks at 0·5, 1·0 and 2 J/kg.

(A conscious child must be anaesthetised or heavily sedated first)

The unconscious child

Coma

Disorder	Common causes
Trauma	• Head injury, child abuse
Seizure	• Overt or subclinical seizures, status epilepticus, postictal state
Infections *(meningo-encephalitis)*	• Bacterial meningitis; *Streptococcus pneumoniae, Haemophilus influenzae, Neisseria meningitidis*, streptococci (group B), *Pseudomonas* species, tuberculosis
	• Viruses; herpes simplex, Japanes Encephalitis Virus (JEV) (in Asia), herpes zoster
	• Mycoplasma
	• Acute spirochitaemia, syphilis, Lyme disease, leptospirosis
	• Parasitic; malarial, rickettsial
	• Cerebral abscess
	• Fungal; *Cryptococcus neoformans*
Metabolic	• Hypoglycaemia (malaria, sepsis in neonates, excess insulin or metabolic disorders)
	• Hyperglycaemia in diabetic ketoacidosis.
	• Hypoxaemia secondary to cardiac/respiratory/septic shock
	• Electrolyte imbalance: hyponatraemia or hypernatraemia
	• Severe dehydration
	• Severe malnutrition
	• Organ failure: liver failure, renal failure, Addison's disease, respiratory failure
	• Drugs: opiates, salicylates, organophosphate, benzodiazepines, thiazides
	• Others; porphyrias, Reye's syndrome
Poisoning	• Alcohol, recreational drugs, accidental/deliberate poisoning
Tumours	• Primary: medulloblastoma, astrocytoma
	• Secondary: leukaemias, sarcomas
Vascular	• Haemorrhage (subdural/subarachnoid), hypertension, hypotension, thrombosis, aortic stenosis, cardiac asystole
	• Vasculitis and collagen vascular syndromes
Systematic inflammatory response syndrome (usually with shock)	• Sepsis, trauma, burns, peritonitis

Focused history

Focus on possible cause, rate of development of unconsciousness, extent of injury, signs of deterioration or recovery, and past medical history.

Examination

Always consider hypoxaemia, hypovolaemia, and hypoglycaemia initially.

Airway and breathing – look, listen, feel

- If responsive to pain only, protect airway and consider early definitive airway to protect lower airways from aspiration.
- Give high flow oxygen.
- Respiratory pattern:
    Irregular due to brainstem lesion or raised intracranial pressure (RICP)
    Rapid due to acidosis or aspirin ingestion
    Slow due to opiate ingestion.

Circulation – HR, capillary refill time (CRT), BP

Pulse: bradycardia may indicate **RICP** or reflect the effects of poisons or drug overdoses.

Blood pressure: hypertensive encephalopathy or **RICP**.

Temperature: sepsis (fever or hypothermia).

Neurological disability – AVPU, pupils, lateralising signs and posturing, followed by specific coma score assessment and full neurological examination

Painful stimuli: supraorbital, nail bed, or sternum.

Pupil size and reactivity: small due to opiate ingestion
                          large due to amphetamine or atropine ingestion
                          unequal/unreactive due to **RICP**.

Posture/oculocephalic reflexes: abnormal in **RICP**.

Neurological examination to establish baseline (tone, power, reflexes, sensation, and coordination where possible).

Identify **RICP** (including herniation syndromes), focal deficits (for example, space occupying lesion (SOL)) and lateralising signs (hemiplegic syndromes).

Further focused examination to identify cause

Skin rashes: infections, for example meningococcal septicaemia, Dengue haemorrhagic fever.

Breath odour: diabetic ketoacidosis, alcohol ingestion, inborn errors of metabolism.

Hepatomegaly: Reye's syndrome, other metabolic disorders.

Fundi: papilloedema, retinal haemorrhages (?shaken baby syndrome).

Glucostix (confirm with lab blood sugar).

Further detailed neurological evaluation

Cranial nerves:
- Pupillary reactions:
  use a bright torch
  consider drugs used, for example opiates.
- Ocular movements:
  eyelid response
  corneal response.
- Oculocephalic reflexes:
  turn the head sharply to one side, eyes move to opposite side in normal
  if eyes only partly deviate or remain fixed then abnormal
  check first no cervical injury.
- Oculovestibular or caloric response:
  Check first no cervical injury. Ascertain the tympanic membrane is intact and no wax.
  tilt the head forward at 30°, instill ice cold water into the ear – the eyes turn to the side of the stimulus in normal brainstem.

Motor function:
- Motor activity, i.e. tremor, multifocal, or none
- Motor response or postures: normal, decerebrate state (extended arms and legs), decorticate state (flexed arms, extended legs), rigidity, hypotonia, extension or flexion of contralateral limbs.

Glasgow Coma Scale (> 4 years)

Activity	Best response	Score
Eye opening	Spontaneous	4
	To verbal stimuli	3
	To pain	2
	None to pain	1
Verbal	Orientated	5
	Confused	4
	Inappropriate words	3
	Non-specific words	2
	None to pain	1
Motor	Follows commands	6
	Localises pain	5
	Withdraws in response to pain	4
	Abnormal flexion (decorticate) to pain	3
	Abnormal extension (decerebrate) to pain	2
	None to pain	1

Adelaide Coma Scale (< 4 years)

Activity	Best response	Score
Eye Opening	Eyes open spontaneously	5
	To request	4
	To voice	3
	To pain	2
	None to pain	1
Verbal	Orientated, alert	5
	Recognisable and relevant words spontaneous cry	4
	Cries only to pain	3
	Moans only to pain	2
	None to pain	1
Motor	Obeys commands	6
	Localises painful stimulus	5
	Withdraws from pain	4
	Abnormal flexion to pain (decorticate)	3
	Abnormal extension to pain (decerebrate)	2
	None to pain	1

Respiratory pattern:
- Irregular: consider seizures
- Cheyne-Stokes: RICP, cardiac failure
- Kussmaul: acidosis, central neurogenic hyperventilation, mid-brain injury, tumour, or stroke
- Apneustic (periodic) breathing: pontine damage, central herniation
- Signs and symptoms of RICP.

Investigations

Essential

1. Clinical chemistry: blood glucose, electrolytes, creatinine, urea, blood gases, liver function tests
2. Blood film for malarial parasites
3. Full blood count, peripheral blood film
4. Septic screen: blood cultures; urinalysis for microscopy, sensitivity and culture; lumbar puncture (LP) in case of high index of suspicion of central nervous system infection. **It should be delayed** if there are:

   features of RICP
   the child is too sick to tolerate the flexed position needed
   infection at puncture site
   bleeding tendency
   and rash of meningococcal septicaemia.

The child should be given antibiotics to cover the possibility of bacterial meningitis.

5. CXR: tuberculosis, severe pneumonia. Further imaging depending on resources available and specific indication. CT or MRI – particularly useful in detecting space-occupying lesions, traumatic injury, contrast dye should be given if an infection or tumour suspected.
6. Toxicology i.e. salicylates, organophosphate, opiates, alcohol, metamphetamines, cannabinoids.
7. Specific metabolic: plasma ammonia and plasma/ CSF lactate; urine/plasma for organic/amino acids.

Management

Immediate (ABC)

- Support respiration if necessary (support ventilation – maintain a PCO_2 of 3·5–5·0 kPa).
- Support circulation to maintain adequate cerebral perfusion (aim to keep systolic BP at normal values for age, avoid hypotension).
- Maintain normo-glycaemia, if blood glucose not available give 5 ml/kg 10% glucose IV or NG.
- Maintain electrolyte balance (avoid hyponatraemia; use 0·9% saline + added glucose NOT 1/5 N dextrose saline). If possible keep serum sodium in high normal range > 135 mmol/l.
- Treat seizures.
- Insert NG tube to aspirate stomach contents.
- Regulate temperature (avoid hyperthermia: that is above 37·5°C).

Treat RICP (see below for more details)

- Mannitol (250–500 mg/kg; that is 1·25–2·5 ml/kg of 20% IV over 15 minutes, and give 2 hourly as required, provided serum osmolality is not > 325 mOsm/L).
- Dexamethasone (for oedema surrounding a space-occupying lesion: 500 micrograms/kg stat and then 50 micrograms/kg every 6 h).
- Catheterisation for bladder care and urine output monitoring.

Intermediate

- Prevent child falling out of bed.
- Nutritional support.
- Skin care, prevent bed sores.
- Eye padding to avoid xerophthalmia.
- Chest physiotherapy to avoid hypostatic pneumonia.
- Restrict fluids to 60% of maintenance if water retention.
- Prevent deep vein thrombosis by physiotherapy.

- Maintain oral and dental hygiene.
- Appropriate care for central and peripheral venous or arterial access to avoid infection.
- Watch for nosocomial infection.

Presenting features of raised intracranial pressure (RICP)

Infants and young children

- Abnormally rapid head growth
- Separation of cranial sutures
- Bulging of anterior fontanelle (usually closes by 18 months)
- Dilatation of scalp veins
- Irritability
- Vomiting
- Loss of truncal tone
- Fluctuating level of responsiveness
- Irregular rate and rhythm of breathing, usually with slowing of respiratory rate and apnoeas – pre-terminal
- Irregular heart rate, usually with bradycardia but occasionally with tachycardia
- Decerebrate attacks (distinguish from epileptic seizures; in decerebrate extends all four limbs and trunk, whereas in seizures flexion of the upper limbs is more usual and there are clear tonic/clonic phases) – pre-terminal
- Unconsciousness is late, often preceded by apnoea – pre-terminal.

Older children

- Headaches
- Vomiting
- Central ataxia
- Failing vision (indicates severe papilloedema)
- Diplopia
- Neck pain and extension — pre-terminal
- Decerebrate attacks — pre-terminal

- Irregular rate and rhythm of breathing, usually with slowing of respiratory rate – pre-terminal
- Irregular heart rate, usually with bradycardia but occasionally with tachycardia, and mounting hypertension with widening pulse pressure – pre-terminal
- Diminishing level of consciousness – pre-terminal.

The absence of papilloedema does not exclude RICP; its presence indicates risk of permanent visual loss.

Management of suspected raised intracranial pressure – RICP

THIS IS A MEDICAL EMERGENCY

- Assess ABC, give high flow oxygen (mask/reservoir 10–15 L/min), and obtain IV/intraosseous access
- Treat shock (see above), if present, but exercise caution with fluid therapy.

DO NOT PERFORM LUMBAR PUNCTURE

- Give mannitol 250 mg/kg to 500 mg/kg IV over 15 minutes (this should be repeated if signs of raised ICP persist). If mannitol is unavailable give frusemide 1 mg/kg IV.

If space-occupying lesion suspected give **dexamethasone by slow IV injection** (500 micrograms/kg stat and then 50 micrograms/kg every 6 h)

Where signs persist despite the above therapy, ideal management would include:

- Rapid sequence induction of anaesthesia and intubation for both airway protection (if GCS < 8 and/or child is unresponsive to painful stimuli) and stabilisation of $P\text{co}_2$.
- Mechanical ventilation with optimal sedation and maintenance of $P\text{co}_2$ within the normal range (ideally between 3·5 and 5 kPa).

Other useful techniques include:

- Placing patient supine with a 30° head-up position
- Avoidance of central venous catheters in internal jugular veins
- Antipyretics to prevent temperatures > 37·5°C
- Full neurological and cardiovascular assessment with regular (at least hourly) assessment of: pupillary responses, conscious level, pulse, blood pressure,

capillary refill time, respiratory rate and effort (pulse oximetry if available) and temperature.

Maintain normoglycaemia and serum sodium (in high normal range > 135 mmol/L)/ osmolality

Monitoring electrolytes, gases, clotting, and full blood count as recommended for shock.

Features of a supratentorial mass lesion

- Dysphasia
- Visual field defects
- Epileptic fits
- Unilateral pupil dilatation indicates a mass ipsilateral to dilated pupil, or on side of pupil that dilated first if bilateral pupillary dilatation.

Management

- Definitive solution is removal of the causative lesion, requires CT and a neurosurgical facility.

Emergency and temporary relief of RICP

As above but also consider:

Infants

Transfontanelle needle tapping of the subdural space, and if there is no subdural effusion, then needle advanced into cerebral ventricle.

Children

Right frontal burr-hole and ventricular drainage

If there is a history of head injury, then "blind" burr-holes when neurosurgical expertise not available and there are unilateral pupillary signs

Allergic reactions and anaphylactic shock

Symptoms	Signs
Mild	
Burning sensation in mouth	Urticarial rash
Itching of lips, mouth, throat	Angio-oedema
Feeling of warmth	Conjunctivitis
Nausea	Red throat
Abdominal pain	
Moderate	
Coughing/wheezing	Bronchospasm
Loose bowel motions	Tachycardia
Sweating	Pallor
Irritability	
Severe	
Difficulty breathing	Severe bronchospasm
Faintness or collapse	Laryngeal oedema
Vomiting	Shock
Uncontrolled defaecation	Respiratory arrest
	Cardiac arrest

Management ABC

- Remove allergen.
- Assess **A**irway:

  give 100% oxygen

  if stridor with obstruction: 10 micrograms/kg epinephrine IM, then 5 ml epinephrine 1 in 1000 nebulised

  if stridor with complete obstruction: intubate or surgical airway

  otherwise consider intubation, call for anaesthetic/ENT assistance.

- Assess **B**reathing:

  if no breathing, 5 rescue breaths with 100% oxygen

  if wheeze, 10 micrograms/kg epinephrine IM

  salbutamol inhaled dose/either 2·5 mg < 5 years or

　　　5·0 mg if > 5 years nebulised with 100% oxygen or
　　　1000 micrograms via spacer (10 × 100 microgram
　　　puffs) + repeated or continuously as required.
- Assess **Circulation**:
　　　if no pulse, start basic life support, assess rhythm and
　　　　treat
　　　if shocked, 10 micrograms/kg epinephrine IM
　　　20 ml/kg 0·9% saline/colloid.

　　*NB: Give epinephrine IM, unless in intractable shock or
　　cardiac arrest when it should be given IV or IO.*

If intubated it can be given at ten times the dose down the
ET tube (that is epinephrine 100 micrograms/kg).
If boluses of epinephrine are ineffective or lasting only a short
time, infusion 0·05–2·0 micrograms/kg/min (preferably via
central vein).

Reassess ABC and continue 100% oxygen
- If airway deterioration, repeat IM epinephrine 10
　micrograms/kg, consider intubation or surgical airway.
- If still wheezy:
　　repeat IM epinephrine 10 micrograms/kg
　　hydrocortisone 4 mg/kg (over 15 minutes) IV
　　aminophylline 5 mg/kg slow IV + 1 mg/kg/h IV infusion
　　　or salbutamol 4–6 microgram/kg slow IV followed by
　　　IV = 0·5–1·0 micrograms/kg/min IV infusion.
- If still shocked:
　　repeat IM epinephrine 10 micrograms/kg
　　20 ml/kg 0·9% saline colloid 4·5% albumin
　　inotropic infusion dopamine or epinephrine: see
　　page 183.
- Asymptomatic:
　　other than rash or itching, oral antihistamine –
　　　chlorpheniramine 250 micrograms/kg (repeat up to
　　　4 times in 24 hours if necessary)
　　oral steroids prednisolone 1·0–2·0 mg/kg total daily
　　　dose (1 month to 12 years).

Status epilepticus

During a seizure

- Place into a left lateral decubitus position (if practical).
- Ensure the AIRWAY IS PATENT and there is ADEQUATE RESPIRATORY function and ADEQUATE CIRCULATORY function.
- If seizure > 5 minutes (or duration unknown) ANTICONVULSANT treatment. Short recurrent seizures should also be treated.
- Treat fever by exposure, tepid sponging, and rectal paracetamol (20 mg/kg).

Investigations

Blood glucose, film for malaria parasites, urea, creatinine, calcium, electrolytes, and full blood count. Urinalysis, BP, lumbar puncture (when meningitis possible, particularly < 2 years), cultures of blood, urine, pharyngeal swab and CSF, relevant X-rays.

Management

- Monitor vital signs (anticonvulsants can cause hypotension and respiratory depression).
- If seizures not controlled by anticonvulsant, general anaesthesia (for example, thiopentone) and muscle relaxants with respiratory support if available.

Diazepam IV/IO 100–250 micrograms/kg Rectal 500 micrograms/kg	or	**Paraldehyde** rectal/IM dose 0·4 ml/kg	or	**Lorazepam** IV/rectal/IO 50–100 micrograms/kg
Can be repeated once		Can be repeated many times and used with diazepam/lorazepam		Can be repeated once

Seizure > 15 minutes

(> 1 year) **Phenytoin** IV 18 mg/kg bolus over 10–30 minutes Monitor ECG/BP	or	(>1 year or on regular phenytoin) **Phenobarbitone** IV 15–20 mg/kg bolus over 10–30 minutes Monitor respiration/BP

If no more seizures then give maintenance treatment for 48 hours (phenytoin 2·5 mg/kg
12 hourly or phenobarbitone 5 mg/kg/day as a single dose).

Seizure > 40 minutes

Admit to intensive care unit for RSI and anticonvulsant infusions

Midazolam	30–300 micrograms/kg over 5 minutes,
	maintain at 30–300 micrograms/kg/h or
Thiopentone	2–8 mg/kg IV for induction then
	maintain per the response 1–5 mg/kg/h or
Chlormethiazole IV 0·8% solution (8 mg/ml)	1–2 ml/kg (8–16 mg/kg) over 5 minutes then 0·5 ml/kg/h (4–8 mg/kg/h)

Maintenance treatment as above for 48 hours after the end of seizure or last seizure

Poisoning

Symptoms and signs

- Sudden unexplained illness in previously healthy child
- Drowsiness or coma
- Convulsions
- Ataxia
- Tachypnoea
- Tachycardia or flushing
- Cardiac arrhythmia or hypotension
- Unusual behaviour
- Pupillary abnormalities.

Management of poisoning

- Remove poison, for example, wash contaminated skin and eyes with water, remove from enclosed space if fire.
- ABCD.
- Test for hypoglycaemia, if not possible treat 5 ml/kg of 10% glucose IV then 0·1 ml/kg/min to keep blood glucose 5–8 mmol/L.
- Treat convulsions with diazepam 100–250 micrograms/kg IV over 5 minutes or 500 micrograms/kg per rectum.
- If opiate overdose suspected give naloxone, 10 micrograms/kg IV repeated up to a maximum of 2 mg (has short half-life therefore infusion of 10–20 micrograms/kg/min may be required).
- Identify the substance ingested or inhaled if possible.

Questions to be asked

What potential medicines, domestic products, berries, plants or animals (snakes, spiders, scorpions, fish) might the patient have had exposure to?

- How much has been taken?
- Earliest possible ingestion time?
- Is the container or a sample available?
- Are other children involved?
- What symptom(s)?
- Use National Poisons Information Centres or computer based references to get information about the side effects, toxicity, and treatment needed.
- Remove, absorb, or neutralise ingested substance immediately.

If corrosive, may be serious risk of injury to the mouth, throat, airway, oesophagus, or stomach. The most dangerous are NaOH or KOH cleaning fluids. Others include bleach and other disinfectants. Serious oesophageal injury with perforations and mediastinitis and later strictures may result.

- The presence of burns within the mouth is of concern and suggests that oesophageal injury is possible.
- Stridor suggests laryngeal damage. NO EMETIC SHOULD BE GIVEN. MILK OR WATER GIVEN AS SOON AS POSSIBLE WILL HELP.

If available, endoscopy may be helpful. A ruptured oesophagus will lead to mediastinitis and should be treated with gastrostomy and prophylactic antibiotics (cefuroxime and metronidazole).

For all poisons except heavy metals and corrosives give activated charcoal (1 g/kg in water). Repeat after 4 hours if a sustained release drug has been taken. If charcoal is not available and life threatening drug such as iron or tricyclic antidepressant, give paediatric ipecacuanha (10 ml for those aged 6 months to 2 years and 15 ml for > 2 years plus a glass of water) to induce vomiting.

*Do not give ipecac if the child has impaired
consciousness, if corrosive solutions have been ingested,
or if kerosene, turpentine or petrol have been ingested
and could be inhaled producing lipoid pneumonia.*

astric lavage with (15 ml/kg of water or 0·9% saline) a wide
ore orogastric tube indicated only if life threatening poison
nd airway is protected. Never for hydrocarbons or corrosives.

Never give salt to induce vomiting.

If laboratory services are available take samples of blood,
vomit, or urine for drug levels as indicated. If comatosed,
check blood glucose and blood gases.

Give antidote if this is indicated for the specific poison.

Admit if ingested iron, pesticides, corrosives, paracetamol,
salicylate, narcotic drugs, or tricyclic antidepressant drugs.

Admit all who have deliberately taken poisons.

Remember someone may have given a child drugs/poisons
intentionally.

Commonly ingested drugs

Local medicines in disadvantaged countries

sually given for diarrhoea and vomiting. May give profound
cidosis, respiratory distress and paralytic ileus.

reatment – treat metabolic disturbance and pass NG tube.

on

M TO REMOVE AS MUCH AS POSSIBLE BY VOMITING or
astric lavage with wide bore orogastric tube.

esferrioxamine 1 g < 12 years and 2 g > 12 years by deep IM
jection repeated every 12 hours until serum iron is normal.

If very ill, give IV infusion of desferrioxamine 15 mg/kg/h to a maximum dose of 80 mg/kg in 24 hours.

Paracetamol

Give charcoal and if possible measure paracetamol level.
N acetylcysteine or methionine immediately to large overdose

If conscious and within 8 hours of ingestion, give methionine orally (under 6 years 1 g every 4 hours for 4 doses; > 6 years 2·5 g every 4 hours for 4 doses).

If child presents > 8 hours after ingestion or cannot be given oral preparation, give IV acetylcysteine (initially as loading dose 150 mg/kg in 200 ml 5% dextrose in 15 minutes, then I infusion of 50 mg/kg in 500 ml 5% dextrose over 4 hours, finally 100 mg/kg in 1 litre 5% dextrose over 16 hours – that a total of 300 mg/kg over 20 hours).

Alcohol

ABCD
Treat hypoglycaemia and hypothermia.

Benzodiazepines

Flumazenil slow IV 10 micrograms/kg. Repeat 1 minute intervals to max 40 micrograms/kg (total maximum dose = 2 mg). If necessary followed by infusion 2–10 micrograms/kg/h.

Salicylates

Acidotic-like breathing, vomiting, and tinnitus with hyperventilation if severe. Fever may occur, peripheral vasodilatation and moderate hyperglycaemia.

Induce vomiting. There is delayed gastric emptying and therefore induce vomiting even if > 4 hours. Also give activated charcoal (1 g/kg and repeat after 4 hours). Sodium bicarbonate 1 mmol/kg IV over 4 hours to correct acidosis and help excrete salicylate. Give sufficient IV fluids to compensate for hyperventilation and give sufficient glucose to minimise ketosis, but regularly monitor blood glucose. Watch electrolytes carefully and avoid hypokalaemia and hypernatraemia. Vitamin K 10 mg IM/IV. In very severe cases, exchange transfusion or haemodialysis if available.

Tricyclic antidepressants

Drowsiness, ataxia, dilated pupils, and tachycardia. Severe poisoning results in cardiac arrhythmias (particularly ventricular tachycardia) and severe hypotension and convulsions. Induce vomiting, perform gastric lavage, and administer charcoal as above BUT CARE WITH AIRWAY IF DROWSY.

Treat convulsions. Monitor the ECG continuously. Give bicarbonate IV. Arrhythmias can be reduced by using IV phenytoin. Loading dose is 15 mg/kg over 20 minutes followed after 12–24 hours by oral maintenance of 2·5–5 mg/kg 12 hourly.
Prolonged cardiac massage may keep child alive long enough for drug to wear off.

Poisonous household and natural products

Bleach: 3–6% sodium hypochlorite
DO NOT INDUCE VOMITING
Treatment – liberal fluids and milk.

Corrosive agents
Oven cleaners (30% caustic soda), kettle descalers (concentrated formic acid), dishwashing powders (silicates and metasilicates), drain cleaners (sodium hydroxide), car battery acid (concentrated sulphuric acid). Symptoms – considerable tissue damage of skin, mouth, oesophagus, or stomach, late strictures may occur.

Treatment – DO NOT INDUCE VOMITING, wash skin and mouth to dilute corrosive plus milk.

Petroleum compounds such as kerosene, turpentine, and petrol

DO NOT INDUCE VOMITING

If inhaled can produce hydrocarbon pneumonia leading to
a cough, respiratory distress with hypoxaemia due to
pulmonary oedema and lipoid pneumonia.

If ingested may cause encephalopathy.

Additional inspired oxygen and possibly steroids
(hydrocortisone 4 mg/kg IV 12 hourly).

Organophosphorus compounds

Insecticides such as DDT and lindane, malathion, chlorthion,
parathion, TEPP, and phosdrin can be absorbed through the
skin, lungs, or ingested. Symptoms resulting from excessive
parasympathetic effects due to inhibition of cholinesterase,
include excessive salivation, lacrimation, bradycardia,
sweating, gastrointestinal cramps, vomiting, diarrhoea,
convulsions, blurred vision and small pupils, muscle
weakness and twitching progressing to paralysis, loss of
reflexes and sphincter control.

Treatment aim is to get rid of poison from:

Eyes – copious irrigation.

Skin – remove contaminated clothing and wash.

GIT – induce vomiting. Give activated charcoal 1 g/kg and
repeat after 4 hours.

Admit all cases as some effects are late.

In severe cases give **atropine** 50–100 micrograms/kg IV or IM.
May need to be repeated every 15–60 minutes until the skin
becomes flushed and dry, the pupils dilate, and tachycardia
develops. To address neuromuscular sequelae add a specific
cholinesterase re-activator and ideally within 12 hours.

Pralidoxime 25–50 mg/kg diluted with 10–15 ml of water by
IV infusion over 30 minutes. It should produce improved
muscle power in 30 minutes. It can be repeated once or twice
as required.

Lead poisoning

This is usually a chronic form of poisoning. The lead can come from paint, from lead piping, from car batteries. In some cultures substances containing lead can be applied for cosmetic purposes; for example Surma in India.

Early signs are non-specific, for example vomiting, abdominal pain, anorexia. Anaemia is usually present. Prior to encephalopathy with raised intracranial pressure, there may be headaches and insomnia. Peripheral neuropathy may be present. x Rays may show bands of increased density at the metaphyses. Harmful effects on the kidneys result in hypertension, aminoaciduria, and glycosuria. There is a microcytic hypochromic anaemia with punctate basophilia. The diagnosis is made by showing a marked increase in urinary lead after d-penicillamine and elevated blood lead levels.

For lead encephalopathy, use IV infusion of edetate calcium (EDTA) in 250 ml of 5% dextrose 15–20 mg/kg every 6 hours for 5–7 days. A repeat course may be needed 2 weeks later.

Boluses of mannitol 250–500 mg/kg IV over 30–60 minutes for raised ICP whilst the above given.

Carbon monoxide poisoning

ABC. Give 100% oxygen as soon as possible (half-life of CO is 5 hours in room air but 1·5 hours in 100% oxygen). A patient can look pink and be hypoxaemic. Guide duration of O_2 on other clinical signs of hypoxia rather than cyanosis. Pulse oximeters give falsely high readings. Cerebral oedema may develop.

Neonatal emergencies

Fluid and electrolyte balance in the ill neonate

Use in-line infusion chamber/burette to avoid fluid overload

Water requirements

- Start newborn on 60 ml/kg /day of IV 10% dextrose, increasing in daily steps of 20–30 ml/kg/day to a *maximum* of 180 ml/kg/day. In the small for gestational age (SGA) baby begin with 90 ml/kg/day to meet glucose requirements.
- Babies enterally fed but too sick or preterm to breastfeed give breastmilk by orogastric tube:
    Day 1 – 60 ml/kg/day
    Day 2 – 80 to 90 ml/kg/day
    Day 3 – 100 to 120 ml/kg/day
    Day 4 – 120 to 150 ml/kg/day
    Day 5 – 140 to 180 ml/kg/day.
- Monitor fluid intake by weighing daily and recording urine output. Look for signs of fluid overload (oedema) or dehydration. If possible measure plasma electrolytes.

Electrolyte requirements

- Sodium 2·5 mmol/kg/day in term babies. Supplement daily IV 10% glucose allowance with 30% sodium chloride (contains 5 mmol Na^+ per ml) or 23% solution (contains 4 mmol of Na^+/ml). In preterm babies much higher urinary sodium losses may equal 10 mmol/kg/day in those of 29 weeks' gestation or less.
- Sodium supplements commenced on second day of life but if respiratory distress wait until diuresis on third or fourth day.

- Potassium 1–2 mmol/kg/day by adding concentrated potassium chloride to 10% dextrose (add 5 ml of 2 mmol/ml potassium chloride (15% solution) to 1 litre of 10% dextrose or 4 ml of 20% solution (2·7 mmol K^+/ml)).

Hypoglycaemia in the neonate

Increased utilisation and/or decreased production or other causes:

- Perinatal stress (asphyxia, sepsis, shock, hypothermia, respiratory failure).
- Polycythaemia.
- Defects in carbohydrate metabolism (galactosaemia, fructose intolerance, glycogen storage disease).
- Endocrine deficiency (adrenal insufficiency, hypothalamic insufficiency, glucagon deficiency).
- Defects in amino acid metabolism (maple syrup urine disease, proprionic acidaemia, methylmalonic acidaemia, tyrosinaemia).
- Exchange transfusion.
- Increased utilisation of glucose: hyperinsulinism – infants of diabetic mothers.
- Erythroblastosis fetalis.
- Islet cell hyperplasia.
- Beckwith–Weidemann syndrome.
- Insulin producing tumours.
- Maternal beta-agonist tocolytic therapy.
- Abrupt interruption of high glucose infusion.
- Malpositioned umbilical arterial catheter infusing high concentration of glucose into coeliac or mesenteric artery (T11–T12) stimulating insulin release.

Hypoglycaemia in the ill neonate

Decreased production/stores:
- Prematurity
- Small/large for gestational age
- Inadequate caloric intake.

Measure blood glucose when seizures, pronounced hypotonia, or diminished consciousness.
Beware of blaming all signs on "hypoglycaemia".
Remember infection.

When to test

- **Symptomatic infants** (lethargy, poor feeding, temperature instability, respiratory distress, new-onset apnoea/bradycardia, jitteriness, seizures): immediately.
- **Infants at risk:** soon after birth (within 2 hours), then hourly until stable at 2·5 mmol/L (45 mg/dl) or higher. Continue to monitor until feeds well established.
- **Infants with known hypoglycaemia:** during treatment.

Management

Infants at risk but appearing well:

- Initiate early feeding within 1–2 hours after birth with breastmilk or formula only if breastmilk is not available, repeated every 2–3 hours or more often on demand.
- Feeding with 5% dextrose is not recommended in infants with hyperinsulinism because of rebound hypoglycaemia.
- Infants of diabetic mothers are unlikely to develop hypoglycaemia on the second day of life if tests in the first 24 hours are satisfactory.

Infants with symptomatic hypoglycaemia, or unable to feed, or who failed correction of glucose levels with enteral feeding

- Start IV glucose bolus 200 mg/kg over 5 minutes (2 ml/kg of 10% glucose in water). **Remember excess glucose by bolus injections can harm the brain**.
- Follow with maintenance infusion of 10% dextrose at a rate of 5–8 mg/kg/min (3–5 ml/kg/h) (occasionally 12–15 mg/kg/min).
- If further episodes occur, bolus repeated and infusion rate increased by 10–15%.
- Exclude infection.
- When administering boluses, never use high concentrations (> 10%) because of risk of IVH and/or cerebral oedema.
- If infusing concentration > 12·5% use a central venous line or umbilical vein catheter.
- Always decrease IV infusion gradually.
- If no IV access, Hypostop Gel (500 micrograms of glucose per ml) 1–2 ml to the oral mucosa.
- Refractory hypoglycaemia may respond to IV hydrocortisone (5–15 mg/kg/day in 3 divided doses 8 hourly).

If > 7 days old and glucose infusion > 8 mg/kg/min, evaluate for endocrine or metabolic disorder.

Treatment of hypocalcaemia in the neonate

0·1 ml/kg of 10% calcium chloride (note 1 ml of calcium chloride 10% = 3 ml of calcium gluconate 10%).

Jaundice in the ill neonate

Jaundice in the neonate

Units (micromol/l = 17·1 × mg%)

"Physiological jaundice"
Common and does not require treatment or investigation if:
- Not present in first 24 hours
- Well, free of infection without enlarged liver or spleen
- Bilirubin < 300 micromoles/litre (approximately 17 mg/dl) at any stage if term (lower level for preterm)
- Bilirubin peaks at 4–5 days
- Fully resolved at 14 days.

Encourage early, unrestricted demand breastfeeding.

Visual inspection (Kramer), unreliable in black babies:
- Any jaundice detectable: > 90 micromoles/L
- Head and neck only: 70–130 micromoles/L
- Trunk, elbows and knees: 190–310 micromoles/L
- Hands and feet jaundiced: > 300 micromoles/L.

In prolonged jaundice (> 14 days) measure *conjugated* bilirubin level.

Pathological jaundice
- Preterm delivery: lower treatment thresholds.
- Haemolytic disease. Isoimmune (for example, Rh (Rh −ve mother, Rh +ve baby in second or subsequent pregnancies)) or ABO incompatibility (Mother O, baby A, B, or AB) or due to red cell disorders (for example, hereditary spherocytosis or G6PD deficiency).
- Infection. Acquired and congenital infection (for example, rubella, CMV infection), congenital also has rash, hepatosplenomegaly, thrombocytopenia, and some conjugated bilirubin.

- Rarely inborn errors of metabolism (galactosaemia) and congenital hypothyroidism.
- Obstructive jaundice. Rarely < 7 days.

Investigation of jaundice

Jaundice < 24 hours most likely infection or haemolytic disease. Has mother borne previously affected babies or a hereditary haemolytic disorder? Signs of sepsis, hepatomegaly, or haemolytic disease?

- Mother's and baby's ABO and Rh. Save serum to cross-match if exchange transfusion required.
- Direct Coombs' test (if positive = an isoimmune haemolytic anaemia).
- G6PD level.
- FBC and reticulocytes.
- Peripheral blood smear (abnormal red cell morphology and/or fragmented red cell forms suggest a red cell disorder and/or haemolysis).
- Thyroid function and urine for non-glucose reducing substance (possible galactosaemia).

Treatment

In a sick, acidotic baby intervene about 40 micromoles/L below the indicated line.

In infants < 31 weeks initiate phototherapy when the bilirubin approaches 85 micromoles/L per kg birth weight and consider exchange for levels above 170 micromoles/L per kg birth weight.

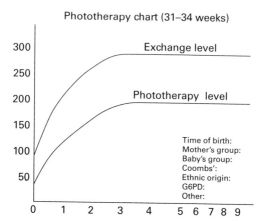

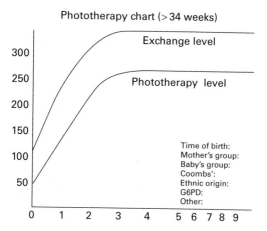

- Tachypnoea – respiratory rate > 60/min
- Retractions (recession)
- Grunting
- SaO_2 will be < 94% in air.

- "Transient tachypnoea" delay in clearing fetal lung fluid (low section Caesarean section (LSCS)).
- Congenital pneumonia or sepsis (often prolonged rupture membranes > 18 hours).
- Surfactant deficiency (also known as "respiratory distress syndrome").
- Pneumothorax.
- Meconium aspiration.
- Congenital abnormalities of the lung or airways (including diaphragmatic hernia).
- Congenital heart disease does **not** cause early respiratory distress. Cyanosis is the more usual presentation; respiratory distress associated with heart failure normally occurs after the first week of life in association with tachycardia, pallor, sweating, hepatomegaly, and excessive weight gain.

Principles of treatment

- Assess oxygenation and give oxygen until pink and SaO_2 94–98%. Avoid hyperoxaemia.
- Arterial blood gas.
- Blood culture and IV antibiotics given. Ampicillin/penicillin and an aminoglycoside (or a third generation cephalosporin).
- Chest x ray.
- Avoid oral feeding: IV 10% glucose (60 ml/kg/day) is safest, peripheral vein or if not possible UVC. If no facilities for IV, breastmilk or 10% glucose (up to 60 ml/kg/day) by orogastric tube.
- Early continuous positive airways pressure (CPAP).
- Intermittent positive pressure ventilation (IPPV).

Causes of neonatal apnoea

- "Apnoea" of prematurity (idiopathic).
- Hypoglycaemia, temperature instability, and anaemia.
- Pulmonary parenchymal disease.
- Airway obstruction (for example, hyperflexion or hyperextension of the neck), especially in premature infants. Congenital airway anomalies (for example, trans-oesophageal fistula (TOF) or "vascular sling").
- Infection. Antibiotics until excluded.
- Seizures.
- Maternal narcotics. Reversed by naloxone (100 micrograms/kg, usually IM), but not if chronic narcotic dependency in pregnancy.

Neonatal infections

- Subtle, non-specific changes in feeding pattern, emesis, irritability, pallor, diminished tone, and/or decreased skin perfusion
- Lethargy, apnoea, tachypnoea, cyanosis, petechiae, and early jaundice
- Fever uncommon, especially with bacterial infection < 7 days
- Temperature instability/hypothermia
- Hypoglycaemia and/or metabolic acidosis.

Maternal risk factors for early onset sepsis

- Maternal chorioamnionitis
- Intrapartum maternal fever (especially 38°C or greater)
- Premature rupture of membranes
- Prolonged rupture of membranes (18 hours or greater)
- Preterm labour
- Maternal bacteriuria (especially β-haemolytic streptococcus)
- Prior infected infant.

Laboratory tests

- Blood culture (about 1ml venous blood)
- WBC and differential poorly predictive of infection. Normal < 48 hours $10-30 \times 10^9$. If $<5 \times 10^9$ or elevated ratio band forms to total neutrophil (mature neutrophils plus bands) (0.3 or greater) supports infection
- Chest x ray
- Lumbar puncture (cytology and culture)
- MSU or suprapubic urine (if onset > 48 hours)
- Blood glucose
- Serum bilirubin if jaundiced.

Management

Stabilise cardiovascular and respiratory systems. Immediate administration of antibiotics (after blood culture):

- Betalactam plus aminoglycoside (ampicillin + gentamicin). Penicillin if ampicillin not available, OR
- Cefotaxime or ceftriaxone (especially gram −ve) some gram +ve need a penicillin derivative.
- Increasing multidrug resistance (ciprofloxacin may be needed).
- Flucloxacillin (IV or oral) if *paronychia, septic spots or umbilical infection*.
- **Give all unwell neonates 1 mg vitamin K IM/IV.**

Meningitis

Presenting features

Include lethargy, irritability, hypotonia, seizures, generalised signs of accompanying sepsis, and a bulging or tense anterior fontanelle. **Always measure and note head circumference**.

Investigations

Lumbar puncture essential. Elevated CSF leucocyte count > 25 cells/mm^3 with a pleocytosis is characteristic. CSF protein in neonatal meningitis may be > 2·0 g/L in a term baby (normal values = < 0·5 g/L) and CSF glucose is typically low (< 1·0 mmol/L or < 30% of blood glucose value). The gram stain may reveal bacteria.

The CSF in preterm babies with IVH can confuse: sometimes there is a mild reactive pleocytosis present for the first few weeks of life. Treat as bacterial meningitis until cultures negative.

If a "bloody tap" is obtained treat as infected and repeat the lumbar puncture after 24 hours.

If a CSF pleocytosis but no organism consider imaging to rule out a parameningeal focus, especially if seizures or focal neurological findings.

Treatment

Betalactam plus aminoglycoside or third generation cephalosporin. Treat for 14 days for gram +ve and 21 days for gram −ve bacteria.

Necrotising enterocolitis

- Treat shock.
- **Stop all enteral feeds** and provide IV fluids, typically 120 ml/kg/day of 10% dextrose with added electrolytes.
- Orogastric tube on low-pressure continuous suction, if available, or leave the tube open with intermittent gastric aspiration (every 4 hours) to keep intestines decompressed.
- Parenteral broad spectrum antibiotics, usually with ampicillin, gentamicin and metronidazole (especially if pneumotosis, perforation, or evidence of peritonitis).
- 1mg vitamin K IV/IM and if bleeding fresh frozen plasma 10 ml/kg.
- Treat for 10–21 days.
- Ideally parenteral nutrition. Enteral feeds (breastmilk) reintroduced slowly at end of therapy (20–30 ml/kg/day) with monitoring of abdomen.

Neonatal seizures

Often subtle (for example, staring, lip smacking/grimacing, deviation of the eyes, cycling movements of limbs); or obvious tonic (extensor) posturing or clonic movements.

Bulging anterior fontanelle suggests intracranial haemorrhage or infection. **Measure head circumference**.

Differential diagnosis

- Hypoxic ischaemic encephalopathy
- Intracranial haemorrhage and cerebral infarction. Always give 1 mg vitamin K IV
- Infection. Exclude/treat meningitis
- Metabolic causes:
    hypoglycaemia
    hypocalcaemia
    hyponatraemia – uncommon unless Na < 120 mmol/L
    hypernatremia – may produce cavernous venous thrombosis. IPA rapid fall or rise in Na more injurious
    pyridoxine dependency (give 50 mg pyridoxine IV during a seizure)
- Kernicterus
- Other rare inborn errors of metabolism (for example, urea cycle defects, non-ketotic hyperglycinaemia) – measure serum amino acids, urine fatty acids, serum lactate and pyruvate, and blood ammonia
- Maternal substance abuse, particularly opiate withdrawal.

Investigations

- Lumbar puncture and blood culture
- Blood glucose, calcium, urea, and electrolytes; blood ammonia if available (arterial)

- Arterial blood gas
- Cranial ultrasound
- Intracranial imaging (head CT if available)
- EEG
- Save urine, plasma, and CSF for metabolic studies.

Treatment

- Stop feeds and give fluids IV.
- Start antibiotics.
- Treat hypoglycaemia if present.
- Monitor heart and respiratory rate, oxygenation (ideally with pulse oximetry), and blood pressure. Treat low SaO_2 or cyanosis with oxygen.
- Consider anticonvulsant therapy: the earlier fits appear, the more frequent they are (more than 2–3/hour), and the longer they last (more than 3 minutes), the more likely this will be required. Fits which interfere with respiration need to be treated. Anticonvulsants can be given as follows:

Phenobarbitone (1st line): 20 mg/kg IV; an additional 10 mg/kg may be required if
  seizures persist or recur

Phenytoin (2nd line): give 20 mg/kg loading dose by slow infusion and monitor for
  hypotension and cardiac arrhythmia

Paraldehyde: rectal, IV or IM 0·2–0·3 ml/kg loading dose and repeat once 4–6 hours
  later

Clonazepam infusion: 100–200 micrograms/kg loading dose (maximum 0·5 mg) then
  10–30 micrograms/kg/h as an infusion (intensive care will be required)

Sodium valproate: 20 mg/kg then 10 mg/kg 12 hourly

Carbamazepine: 2·5 mg/kg 12 hourly

Pyridoxine 100 mg IV (then if seizures stop immediately 50 mg 4 hourly)

Neonatal Hypoxic Ischaemic Encephalopathy (HIE)

Fetal distress such as abnormal cardiotachograph (CTG), cord pH < 7·2, low Apgar score (3 or less at 5 minutes) despite appropriate resuscitation. Multiorgan dysfunction such as oliguria, haematuria (signifying acute tubular necrosis (ATN)), increased transaminase levels (hepatic necrosis), myocardial dysfunction.

Sarnat's clinical grading may help to guide treatment and aid prognosis.

| | Sarnat stage | | |
	Mild (stage 1)	Moderate (stage 2)	Severe (stage3)
Conscious level	Hyperalert	Lethargic	Stuporose
Muscle tone	Normal	Hypotonic	Flaccid
Seizures	Rare	Common	Severe
Feeding	Sucks weakly	Needs tube feeds	Needs tube feeds
Respiration	Spontaneous	Spontaneous	Absent
Prognosis	Good	Guarded	Very bad

Treatment

- Maintain blood gases, blood pressure, and fluid balance.
- Avoid hyponatraemia.
- If acute renal failure (ARF) restrict fluids to 40 ml/kg/day (to reflect insensible losses) and avoid potassium.
- Treat seizures.

Specific emergencies

Upper airway problems

Emergency treatment of croup

Patient will be frightened, so do not stick instruments
in throat or cause pain from repeatedly trying to insert a
venous cannula. Crying increases oxygen demand and
laryngeal obstruction. Keep child on mother's lap. Ask
mother to alert staff if child breathes more quickly or
worse sternal recession develops.

Encourage oral fluids.

If cyanosed or SaO_2 < 94% in air give high flow humidified
oxygen through nasal cannulae or a facemask held just
below nose/mouth by parent. Do not use nasopharyngeal
catheters.

Oral paracetamol for pain.

Dexamethasone 0·6 mg/kg orally. If vomits same dose IM.
Alternative nebulised budesonide 2 mg in 2 ml. It may be
repeated 30–60 minutes later.

If severe obstruction, nebulise epinephrine
(5 ml of 1 in 1000) with oxygen. If effective, repeat 2 hourly
as required. Produces improvement for 30–60 minutes.
Arrange urgently ENT surgeon and anaesthetist.

If intubated, 1 mg/kg prednisilone every 12 hours reduces
duration of intubation.

Severely ill, toxic or with measles, consider bacterial
tracheitis and antibiotic against *Streptococcus pneumoniae,
Haemophilus influenzae,*
and *Staphylococcus aureus*. If available, cefuroxime
150 mg/kg/day in 4 doses IV or cephalexin orally 25 mg/kg
6 hourly. Chloramphenicol 25 g/kg IV or orally 6 hourly
is alternative.

Acute epiglottitis

DO NOT	**DO**
Examine the throat	Reassure and calm the child
Lie child down	Attach pulse oximeter and give warm
x Ray neck	humidified O_2 if SaO_2 < 94% by mask
Perform invasive procedures	held below nose/mouth by mother
Use nasopharyngeal tube O_2	Call ENT surgeon and anaesthetist
Upset child by trying to gain	Gain venous access after
venous access	airway has been protected

Management

- **Elective intubation** under GA. Diagnosis confirmed by laryngoscopy just prior to intubation ("cherry-red epiglottis").
- Whilst anaesthetised: do **blood cultures, throat swab, IV line**.
- Recommended antibiotics: chloramphenicol or cefuroxime or cefotaxime or ceftriaxone immediately IV.
- Following intubation breathe humidified air (or air plus oxygen) spontaneously with CPAP. Sedation (discuss with anaesthetist) to prevent self extubation. Alternatively child arms held onto thorax using a bandage. Most ready for extubation after 48 hours.

Contrasting features of croup and epiglottitis

Feature	Croup	Epiglottitis
Onset:	Over days	Over hours
Preceding coryza:	Yes	No
Cough:	Severe, barking	Absent or slight
Able to drink:	Yes	No
Drooling saliva:	No	Yes
Appearance:	Unwell	Toxic, very ill
Fever:	< 38·5°C	> 38·5°C
Stridor:	Harsh	Soft
Voice:	Rasping	Reluctant to speak, muffled
Intubation needed in:	1%	80%

Acute asthma

For moderate asthma

- Avoid procedures which may exacerbate respiratory distress.
- **Give regular inhaled beta-2 agonist bronchodilator**, for example, salbutamol aerosol 200–1000 micrograms via spacer or 2·5 mg for < 5 years and 5 mg for > 5 years via nebuliser 2–4 hourly (**use oxygen to drive the nebuliser**).
- Give oral prednisolone 0·5 mg/kg (maximum of 40 mg) after food/milk or IV hydrocortisone 4 mg/kg 12–24 hourly.

Severe or life-threatening asthma

Features include

- Too breathless to feed, drink or talk
- Marked recession/use of accessory muscles
- Respiratory rate >50 breaths/min
- Pulse rate >140 beats/min
- Poor chest movement/silent chest
- Exhaustion/agitation/reduced conscious level.

Management

- **ABCD.**
- **100% oxygen** via facemask with reservoir bag at 10–15 L/min. Keep SaO_2 > 94% by facemask or nasal cannulae.
- Inhaled beta-2 agonist **bronchodilator** given **continuously at** first and then 0·5–2 hourly, for example salbutamol aerosol 1–2 mg (10–20 puffs) via spacer, or 2·5–10 mg (depending on severity start at 2·5 mg if < 5 years, 5 mg > 5 years) via nebuliser, and repeated. **Use oxygen to drive nebulisers**.
- If above two methods not available, give subcutaneous epinephrine 10 micrograms/kg (0·01 ml/kg of 1 in 1000) up to a maximum single dose of 0·3 ml using a 1 ml syringe. If no improvement after 20 minutes, repeat dose.
- Prednisolone or hydrocortisone – as under "for moderate asthma" above.

- IV salbutamol (loading dose 5 micrograms/kg over
  5 minutes, followed by 1–5 micrograms/kg/min) by IV
  infusion. Severe and life-threatening hypokalaemia may
  occur with IV salbutamol, potentiated by steroids. Monitor
  the ECG and if available check K^+ regularly (minimum
  12 hourly). Ensure maintenance K^+ intake is given.

or

- Aminophylline (loading dose 5 mg/kg over 20 minutes,
  followed by 1mg/kg/h by IV infusion). Monitor rhythm with
  ECG.

Heart failure

Signs
Tachycardia

Raised jugular venous pressure (*often not seen in infants*)

Lung crepitations on auscultation (most basal)

Gallop rhythm

Enlarged liver

Management
- Beware IV fluids (especially Na^+)
- Give calorie supplements + NG feeding if inadequate
  oral intake.
- Bed rest, semi-upright, legs dependent.
- Oxygen if respiratory distress or hypoxaemia due to
  pulmonary oedema ($SaO_2 < 94\%$ sea level).
- Relieve fever if > 38°C.
- When pulmonary oedema, frusemide 1 mg/kg IV should
  produce diuresis in 2 hours. If ineffective, give
  2 mg/kg IV and repeat after 12 hours if necessary
- Then oral frusemide 1 mg/kg once, twice, or three times
  per day. Dose frequency to control symptoms, PLUS
- Spironolactone 1 mg/kg once, twice, or three times per day
  matching the dose frequency of frusemide to enhance
  diuresis and prevent frusemide related hypokalaemia.

- If frusemide without spironolactone, oral potassium 3–5 mmol/kg/day should be given.
- Captopril up to a maximum of 1 mg/kg × 3/day (following 100 micrograms/kg test dose) if more than twice daily diuretics are needed.

Endocarditis prophylaxis

See table on page 72. If allergic to penicillin or the child has had more than one dose of penicillin in the last month substitute another antibiotic in place of amoxicillin, for example:

- 50 mg oral clindamycin for every 250 mg oral amoxicillin that would have been given
- 75 mg of IV clindamycin for every 250 mg of IV amoxicillin that would have been given or
- 20 mg/kg IV vancomycin (max. 1 g) in place of IV amoxicillin.

Management of acute rheumatic fever

- Bed rest during acute phase.
- Eradicate streptococcal infection (oral penicillin V 12·5 mg/kg 6 hourly for 10 days).
- Commence aspirin 90–120mg/day in 4 divided doses. **Reduce the dose to two-thirds when clinical response. When the creative protein (CRP)/erythrocyte sedimentation rate (ESR) normalises, taper the aspirin dose over 2 weeks.**
- Give prednisolone 2 mg/kg/day (max. 60 mg/day) in place of aspirin if carditis or pericarditis. Give for 3 weeks then taper dose over a further 2–3 weeks. As prednisolone dose falls, commence aspirin 50 mg/kg/day in 4 divided doses and stop aspirin 1 week after prednisolone is stopped.
- Treat heart failure.

   Urgent valve replacement sometimes required.

- Endocarditis prophylaxis is needed after carditis.
- For chorea, haloperidol (12·5–25 micrograms/kg twice daily – maximum 10 mg/day < 12 years, 6o mg/day > 12 years).

	< 5 years old	5–10 years old	< 10 years old
Dental or surgical procedures under local anaesthetic	Oral amoxicillin 750 mg 1 hour before procedure	Oral amoxicillin 1-5g 1 hour before procedure	Oral amoxicillin 3 g 1 hour before procedure
Dental or surgical procedures under general anaesthetic	IV amoxicillin 250 mg on induction + oral amoxicillin 125 mg 6 hours later	IV amoxicillin 500 mg on induction + oral amoxicillin 250mg 6 hours later	IV amoxicillin 1 g on induction + oral amoxicillin 500 mg 6 hours later
High risk cases (prosthetic valve/previous endocarditis/ genitourinary procedure)	IV amoxicillin 250 mg + IV gentamicin 2 mg/kg on induction + oral amoxicillin 125 mg 6 hours later	IV amoxicillin 500 mg + IV gentamicin 2 mg/kg (max 120 mg) on induction + oral amoxicillin 250 mg 6 hours later	IV amoxicillin 1 g + IV gentamicin 2 mg/kg (max 120 mg) on induction + oral amoxicillin 500 mg 6 hours later

To prevent recurrence IM benzathine penicillin 1·2 MU once a month or oral penicillin V or erythromycin up to 1 year 62·5 mg, 1–5 years 125 mg, 6–12 years 250 mg and > 12 years 500 mg ALL twice per day after the acute attack (for life).

Features suggesting cause of central cyanosis in an infant

Cardiac	**Respiratory**
Term baby	Premature
Mild tachypnoea but no respiratory distress	Respiratory distress
May have cardiac signs on examination	Chest x ray: abnormal lung fields
Arterial blood gas $Po_2\downarrow$, $Pco_2\downarrow$ or normal	Arterial blood gas $Po_2\downarrow$, $Pco_2\uparrow$ or normal
Fails hyperoxia test	Passes hyperoxia test

The hyperoxia test

- Ensure good IV access
- Monitor oxygen saturations continuously
- Give 100% oxygen for 10 minutes
- Take an arterial blood gas in the right arm (preductal)
- If PO_2 < 20 kPa (150 mmHg), a cardiac cause of cyanosis is likely (the test is "failed")
- If PO_2 > 20 kPa (150 mmHg), a respiratory cause of cyanosis is likely (the test is "passed")
- SaO_2 (pulse oximetry) < 80% baseline and SaO_2 < 90% after 10 minutes in 100% O_2 suggests cyanotic heart defect
- **Oxygen rarely closes arterial duct, precipitating profound hypoxaemia**
- Prostaglandin E (which opens the duct) should be available (starting dose = 10 nanograms/kg/min)

Features that help to distinguish the three types of cyanotic heart defect

	Low pulmonary blood flow	Complete transposition of great arteries (TGA)	Common mixing lesion
Po_2 at rest	Often ≤ 35 mmHg	Often ≤ 35 mmHg	Often ≥ 45 mmHg
Sao_2 at rest	< 80%	< 80%	80–90%
Po_2 hyperoxia test	Often ≤ 50 mmHg	Often ≤ 50 mmHg	75–200 mmHg
Sao_2 hyperoxia	< 90%	< 90%	90–100%
Chest x ray	Reduced pulmonary vascular markings	Normal or increased pulmonary vascular markings ± narrow mediastinum	Normal or increased pulmonary vascular markings

Acute gastroenteritis

Signs – unreliable in severe malnutrition

No dehydration (< 3% weight loss)	Mild dehydration (3–5% weight loss)	Moderate dehydration (6–9% weight loss)	Severe dehydration (10+% weight loss)
	Increased thirst	Loss of skin turgor, tenting when pinched	More pronounced effects seen than in moderate dehydration. Lack of urine output
NO SIGNS	Slightly dry mucous membranes	Sunken eyes. Sunken fontanelle in infants	Hypovolaemic shock, including: a rapid and feeble pulse (the radial pulse may be undetectable), low or undetectable blood pressure (very late sign), cool and poorly perfused extremities
		Restless or irritable behaviour	Over sternum, decreased capillary refill > 2 seconds, and peripheral cyanosis. Rapid, deep breathing (acidosis). Altered consciousness or coma
		Dry mucous membranes	

- Weigh child or use child's age to estimate dehydration.
- Look for abdominal mass or distension.
- In neonate beware sepsis.
- Be aware typhoid, surgical conditions (for example, intussusception), antibiotic associated colitis, and irritable bowel disease (rare).

Management

Two phases: rehydration and maintenance. In both, excess fluid losses must be replaced continuously.

Fluid deficit

No signs of dehydration: < 5% fluid deficit = < 50 ml/kg
Some dehydration: 5–9% fluid deficit = 50–90 ml/kg
Severe dehydration: > 10% fluid deficit = >100 ml/kg.

Rehydration therapy based on degree of dehydration. USE ReSoMal (lower Na content) instead of standard ORS (oral rehydration solution) in children with severe malnutrition.

Mild dehydration (3–5% fluid deficit)

- Commence ORAL REHYDRATION with 50 ml/kg over 2–4 hours.
- Parent gives small amounts (for example, one teaspoon) of solution containing 50–90 mEq/L of sodium (for example, oral rehydration solution (ORS)) frequently.
- Gradually increase amount, as tolerated, using teaspoon, syringe, medicine dropper, cup, or glass.
- REASSESS HYDRATION after 2–4 hours, then progress to the maintenance phase or continue rehydration.

Moderate dehydration (6–9% fluid deficit)

ORS 100 ml/kg, given over 2–4 hours.

Severe dehydration (≥ 10% fluid deficit, shock)

- IV REHYDRATION IMMEDIATELY. Give ORS enterally (oral or N/G) until drip set up (2 IV lines if possible) or even cut down, femoral venous or intraosseous lines.
- Give boluses 10–20 ml/kg IV of Hartmann's solution (page 187) (Na = 131 mmol/L; K = 5 mmol/L; HCO_3 = 29 mmol/L; Ca = 2 mmol/L) until pulse, perfusion (CAPILLARY REFILL), and mental status return to normal. The concentration of potassium is low and there is no glucose to prevent hypoglycaemia. This is especially important in infants and young children and can be corrected by adding 100 ml of

50% glucose to 500 ml of Hartmann's giving approximately a 10% glucose solution (adding 50 ml gives a 5% solution).

If Hartmann's is not available, 0·9% saline. However it does not contain a base to correct acidosis and does not replace potassium losses (therefore add KCl 5 mmol/L). Also add dextrose as above.

- DO NOT USE hypotonic IV solutions such as 5% glucose or 0–18% saline plus 4% glucose WHICH ARE DANGEROUS IF GIVEN QUICKLY (HYPONATRAEMIA AND CEREBRAL OEDEMA).

- Usually 100 ml/kg of IV replacement fluids (Hartmanns or 0·9% saline plus KCl) is required and usually given as follows:

Age	First give 30 ml/kg in	Then give 70 ml/kg in
Infants (under 12 months)	1 hour*	5 hours
Older child	30 minutes*	2·5 hours

* Repeat once if shock is still present.

- When level of consciousness normal, give remaining deficit enterally as ORS.
- Reassess regularly.
- Continue breastfeeding.

All children should start to receive ORS solution (about 5 ml/kg/h) when they can drink without difficulty, which is usually within 3–4 hours (for infants) or 1–2 hours (for older patients). This provides additional base and potassium, which may not be adequately supplied by IV fluid.

Hypernatraemia (Na >150 mmol/L)

Results from child given hypertonic drinks with too high sugar (for example, soft drinks, commercial fruit drinks) or salt. Thirst out of proportion to other signs of dehydration.

Convulsions when Na > 165 mmol/L, and especially when IV therapy. Seizures less likely when treated with ORS. IV rehydration must **not** lower Na too rapidly. Correct over at least 48 hours. IV glucose solutions are particularly dangerous: can result in cerebral oedema.

Hyponatraemia (Na < 130 mmol/L)

From child being given mostly water, or watery drinks containing little salt. Common in shigellosis and severe malnutrition with oedema. Causes lethargy and, less often, seizures. ORS solution is safe and effective for hyponatraemia: except in malnutrition/oedema, where standard ORS contains too much sodium; use ReSoMal if available or diluted ORS.

Hypokalaemia (K < 3 mmol/L)

Inadequate replacement of K especially in malnutrition. Causes muscle weakness, paralytic ileus, impaired kidney function, and cardiac arrhythmias. Hypokalaemia is worsened when base (bicarbonate or lactate) is given to treat acidosis without simultaneously providing potassium. Deficit corrected by ORS and foods rich in potassium during diarrhoea and after it has stopped (bananas, coconut water, dark green leafy vegetables).

If K^+ < 2.0 mmol/L or ECG signs (= flat T waves) then give IV infusion of KCl carefully at a rate of 0.2 mmol/kg/h with serum K^+ checked after 3 hours. Potassium for injection MUST be diluted before use and thoroughly mixed before being given. *The maximum infusion rate is 0.5 mmol/kg/h of potassium.*

Injectable KCl usually contains 1.5 g, that is 20 mmol of potassium in 10 ml, and can be given orally. The daily requirement of K^+ is 2–3 mmol/kg.

Replacement of ongoing fluid losses

10 ml/kg or in older children a cup or small glass of ORS for each watery or loose stool passed, and 2 ml/kg of fluid for each vomit.

USE either low-sodium ORS (containing 40–60 mEq/L of sodium) or ORS containing 75–90 mEq/L of sodium with an additional source of low-sodium fluid (for example, breastmilk, formula, or clean water).

Oedematous eyelids usually indicate over-rehydration but may indicate malnutrition. If this develops, stop ORS, and give breastmilk, plain water, and food. Do not give diuretic. When the oedema has gone, resume ReSoMaL or low Na^+ ORS.

	WHO ORS bicarbonate solution	Low Na^+ ORS solution (for example Dioralyte)	ReSoMal
Na^+	90	60	45
K^+	20	20	40
Cl^-	80	60	
HCO_3^-	30		
Citrate		10	
Glucose	111	90	125 mmol/L

Home made ORS: to 1 litre clean water, add

8 level teaspoons sugar

1 level teaspoon salt

Fruit juice for taste

Severe malnutrition

Principles of treatment

Phase 1 (1–7 days)	Transition (3–4 days)	Phase 2 (usually 14–21 days)
Treat or prevent dehydration, hypoglycaemia, hypothermia		
Treat infection	Treat helminths	

Continued

Phase 1 (1–7 days)	Transition (3–4 days)	Phase 2 (usually 14–21 days)
Correct electrolyte imbalance		
Do NOT give iron	Do not give iron	Correct nutrient deficiencies and iron deficiency
DIET: maintenance intake	Moderate intake	High food intake
Stimulate child	Stimulate child	Stimulate child Provide physical activities Prepare for discharge

General points

- Protect from infections in warm room (25–30°C) without draughts.
- Wash minimally and with warm water and immediately dry.
- Mother to stay with child, especially at night.
- Avoid IV infusions as high risk of heart failure. Only indication is unconsciousness due to circulatory collapse. Only indication for blood transfusion is when anaemia is life threatening.
- IV cannulae removed immediately after treatment.
- NG feeding if:
    anorexia with intake of < 70 kcal/kg
    severe dehydration with inability to drink
    cannot drink and eat because of weakness or clouded consciousness
    painful or severe mouth or oesophageal lesions (herpes, candida, cancrum oris)
    repeated, very frequent vomiting
    try not to tube feed for > 3–4 days; try to breastfeed or feed by mouth as much as possible.

Dehydration with severe malnutrition

Not the same as in non-malnourished child (with exception of cholera).

Signs to assess dehydration unreliable in severe malnutrition. *Assume all children with acute watery diarrhoea have some dehydration*.

Specifically:

- history and observation of frequent WATERY diarrhoea
- history of recent sinking of the eyes: the eyes appear "staring"
- History of not passing urine for 12 hours
- History and observation of thirst.

Reduced skin turgor and sunken eyes (longstanding) are features of malnutrition. Similar appearance can be caused by toxic shock with dilatation of blood vessels – these patients should not be treated as simply dehydrated.

Standard WHO-ORS solutions have too high sodium and too low potassium for children with severe malnutrition. Use ReSoMal (rehydration solution for malnutrition).

Children with watery diarrhoea in an adequate clinical state:
At admission, one dose of ReSoMal orally or NG and feed with phase 1 diet. Further ReSoMal after each stool or vomit.

50 ml for children less than 85 cm in length (approximately < 2 years)
100 ml for children over 85 cm in length (> 2 years).

If ReSoMal not available modify ORS as below.

Children with watery diarrhoea in a poor clinical state:
ReSoMal 10 ml/kg per hour for first 2 hours and then 5 ml/kg per hour until rehydration is complete. (Slower than normally nourished children.)

ReSoMal
Na = 45 mmol/L
K = 40 mmol/L
Mg = 3 mmol/L
Glucose = 125 mmol/L

Rehydration is complete when child is alert, no longer thirsty, and has passed urine. There should be less sunken eyes and fontanelle and improved skin turgor (note: loss of sunken eyes may be a sign of overhydration, development or exacerbation of oedema is sign of excess fluid administration).

70 ml of ReSoMal per kg of weight per day is usually enough to restore hydration. However, rehydration can quickly lead to fluid overload with cardiac failure or sudden death. Malnourished children cannot excrete excess sodium. Assess every 30 minutes during the first 2 hours then every hour. weigh twice daily.

Mark edge of liver on the skin with marker pen at start of rehydration.

ReSoMal should also be stopped immediately if:

Body weight increases by 10% or more
Liver edge increases > 2 cm
Respiratory or pulse rate increase
Jugular veins become engorged
Oedema appears or eyelids become puffy.

Breastfeeding should continue during rehydration. Phase 1 diet should start immediately when child is alert. If severe dehydration, feeding should start as soon as alert and treated (2–3 hours).

When no commercial ReSoMal is available:

To **2 litres** of clean boiled/filtered water add:

1 bag of Standard ORS (WHO)
50 g of sugar
1 dose of mineral/vitamin mix (6·5 g)

(note this is double the quantity of water that is normally used – 2 litres so solution is half strength).

Emergency treatment of severe dehydration by IV infusion

Only where shock clouds consciousness: alert children should never get infusion.

Severe dehydration and septic shock are difficult to differentiate.

- Eyelid retraction with history of diarrhoea is sign of severe dehydration. In septic shock eyelids droop.
- If unconscious (or asleep) without eyelids together, dehydration or hypoglycaemia (a sign of excess adrenalin) is present.
- Superficial veins may be dilated in septic shock: always constricted in severe dehydration.

Immediate treatment:

- Give 15 ml/kg IV over 1 hour of Hartmann's solution with 5% glucose, or 0·9% saline with 5% glucose.
- At same time, insert NG tube and give ReSoMal 10 ml/kg per hour.
- Monitor carefully for overhydration: check respiratory rate every 15 minutes.

If after 1 hour the child is improving but still severely dehydrated continue NG ReSoMal 10 ml/kg/h for up to 5 hours.

If after 1 hour the child has not improved assume septic shock and treat.

Electrolyte problems in severe malnutrition

All have deficiencies of potassium and magnesium which may take > 2 weeks to correct. Do not treat oedema with diuretic.

Excess body sodium exists even though the plasma sodium may be low. **Do not give high sodium loads. Prepare food without adding salt**.

- Give extra potassium (3–4 mmol/kg daily)
- Give extra magnesium (0·4–0·6 mmol/kg daily).

Infection in severe malnutrition

Presume all have infection. Clinical signs may be absent.
Give broad spectrum antibiotics to all plus specific antibiotics
for identified organisms.

No specific infection and no suspected septic shock

Give broad spectrum antibiotics according to local resistance
on admission to all children with severe malnutrition.

- amoxicillin/ampicillin (50 mg/kg IV 6 hourly for 2 days
  then orally 50 mg/kg 6 hourly for 5 days) plus gentamicin
  7·5 mg/kg IV once daily for 7 days.

If fails to improve after 48 hours:

- Add chloramphenicol 50 mg/kg load then 25 mg/kg
  6 hourly IV/IM/oral, or
- Cefotaxime 50–100 mg/kg IV/IM 8 hourly or ceftriaxone
  50–100 mg/kg IV/IM 24 hourly.
- Metronidazole 7·5 mg/kg orally 8 hourly for 7 days is
  frequently also given.

Septic shock: emergency treatment

- Clouding of consciousness
- Rapid respiratory rate:
    - > 50 breaths/min for children from 2 to 12 months
    - > 40 breaths/min for children from 12 months to 5 years
- Rapid pulse rate
- Cold hands and feet with visible subcutaneous veins
- Signs of dehydration but without a history of watery
  diarrhoea
- Hypothermia or hypoglycaemia
- Poor or absent bowel sounds
- An abdominal splash when the child is shaken.

*Difficult to distinguish between severe dehydration and
septic shock in severe malnutrition*

If circulatory collapse

Give 20 ml/kg IV of 0·9% saline then treat as for severe dehydration by IV infusion of 15 ml/kg Hartmann's with 5% glucose over 1 hour.

- Broad spectrum antibiotics (ampicillin + gentamicin) immediately (see above)
- Warm the child to prevent or treat hypothermia
- Feeding and fluid maintenance by NG or orally.

Hypothermia: prevention and treatment

Rectal or oral < 35·5°C (with low reading thermometer). In severe malnutrition thermoneutral air temperature is 28–32°C. At 24°C can become hypothermic. Those with infection or extensive skin lesions at particular risk. A hypothermic, malnourished child should always be assumed to have septicaemia.

Prevention

Cover with clothes and blankets plus warm hat.
Ensure mother sleeps with child. Do not leave child alone in bed at night.
Keep the ward closed during night.
Avoid wet nappies, clothes, or bedding.
Do not wash very ill children. Others to be washed quickly with warm water and dried immediately.
Feed frequently. Ensure feeds occur during the night.
Avoid medical examinations that leave the child cold.

Emergency treatment

Immediately place on the caretaker's bare chest or abdomen (skin to skin) and cover both of them. Give mother a hot drink to increase her skin blood flow.
If no adult available clothe well (including head) and put near a lamp/heat source.
Immediately treat for hypoglycaemia and then start normal feeds.
Give broad spectrum antibiotics.
Monitor rectal temperature until normal (> 36·5°C).

Hypoglycaemia: prevention and treatment

Blood glucose < 3·0 mmol/L. If cannot be measured, assume hypoglycaemia:

- Lethargy, limpness, loss of consciousness, or convulsions
- Drowsiness/unconsciousness with the eyelids partly open, or retraction of the eyelids
- Low body temperature (< 36·5°C).

Sweating and pallor do **not** usually occur.

Prevention

Frequent small feeds (day and night)
Feeding should start while child is being admitted
Treat infections.

Emergency treatment

If can drink give therapeutic milk or 50 ml of glucose 10%, or 50 ml of drinking water plus 10 g of sugar (1 teaspoon of sugar in 3·5 tablespoons of clean water). Follow this with the first feed as soon as possible. If achievable, divide first feed into 4 and give half hourly. If not, give whole feeds every 2 hours during day and night.

If unconscious or convulsing give 5 ml/kg glucose 10% IV and/or if IV is not possible give 5 ml/kg of glucose 10% by NG tube. Continue frequent feeding. Give broad spectrum antibiotics. If convulsions exclude cerebral malaria, meningitis/encephalitis, thiamine deficiency, hypernatraemic/hyponatraemic dehydration (especially in hot dry climates). If blood glucose available and is low, repeat after 30 minutes.

Congestive heart failure (see page 70)

Common and dangerous usually several days after admission. During early recovery from severe malnutrition, sodium mobilised from tissues before kidney recovers to excrete excess. All blood transfusions must therefore be done as soon as possible (within 1–2 days of admission).

Usually caused by

- Misdiagnosis of dehydration with consequent inappropriate "rehydration".
- Very severe anaemia.
- Overload due to blood transfusion (consider exchange transfusion).
- A high sodium diet, using conventional ORS, or excess ReSoMal.
- Inappropriate treatment of "re-feeding diarrhoea" with re-hydration solutions.

Excess weight gain is the most reliable sign – daily weights should be taken on all malnourished children. If weight rises, especially if > 5%, diagnose heart failure, if weight is lost diagnose pneumonia.

Signs

- Fast breathing
    - > 50 breaths/min for children from 2 to 12 months
    - > 40 breaths/min for children from 12 months to 5 years
- Lung crepitations
- Respiratory distress
- Tachycardia
- Engorgement of the jugular veins
- Cold hands and feet
- Cyanosis or SaO_2 < 94% in air at sea level
- Hepatomegaly (see above) or increase in liver by > 2 cm.

Emergency treatment

Stop all intake and IV fluid. No fluid until cardiac function improved, even if takes 24–48 hours. Frusemide IV (1 mg/kg). If potassium intake assured (F100 has adequate potassium) then give single dose of digoxin ORALLY (20 micrograms/kg).

Measles: prevention and treatment in severe malnutrition

All > 6 months vaccinated on admission, second dose at
   discharge.

Isolate any suspected cases.

Review vaccination status of all patients in the ward.

Give two doses vitamin A (see below) separated by
   1 day.

Micro-nutrient deficiencies in severe malnutrition

Daily multivitamin supplement.

Zinc 2 mg/kg/day, copper 0·3 mg/kg/day combined with
   potassium and magnesium to make an electrolyte/
   mineral solution which is added to ReSoMal and
   to feeds.

AVOID iron during the first 2 weeks until the child is gaining
   weight.

In goitrous regions, potassium iodide should be added to
   mineral mixture (12 mg/2500 ml) or give Lugol's iodine
   5–10 drops per day.

Vitamin A deficiency: prevention and treatment

Routine preventive treatment

One dose of vitamin A.

Weight	Dose at admission
< 6 kg	50 000 IU once
6–10 kg	100 000 IU once
> 10 kg	200 000 IU once

Treatment of xerophthalmia or measles

Three doses of Vitamin A treatment given.

Weight	Dosage		
	Day 1	Day 2	Day 14
< 6 kg	50 000 IU	50 000 IU	50 000 IU
6–10 kg	100 000 IU	100 000 IU	100 000 IU
> 10 kg	200 000 IU	200 000 IU	200 000 IU

If eyes inflamed or ulcerated:

- Instil chloramphenicol or tetracycline eye drops, 2–3 hourly as required for 7–10 days.
- Instil atropine eye drops, 1 drop 3 times daily for 3–5 days.
- Cover with saline-soaked eye pads.
- Bandage eye(s).

Note: Children with vitamin A deficiency are photophobic and have eyes closed. Examine very gently to prevent corneal rupture.

Iron deficiency and anaemia treatment

5 mg of folic acid on admission, then 1 mg/day. Iron should never be given during phase I or transition phase. Oral iron supplement should start 14 days after admission. One crushed tablet of ferrous sulphate (200 mg) to 2 litres of therapeutic milk or ferrous sulphate 3 mg/kg/day.

Emergency treatment of very severe anaemia

Blood transfusion is potentially dangerous. Aim for partial exchange transfusion.

Indicators:

- Hb < 4 g/100 ml
- With signs of heart failure due to anaemia (at immediate risk of death).

Transfuse 10 ml per kg of packed cells (or whole blood). Continuously observe cannula in an artery or central vein, possibly also a vein in the antecubital fossa.
2·5 ml/kg of anaemic blood is first removed and then 5 ml/kg of appropriately screened and cross-matched blood is

transfused, 2·5 ml/kg is again taken and the cycle repeated.
**If partial exchange not possible and heart failure present,
give 10 ml/kg ideally as packed cells otherwise as whole
blood. Transfuse over 4 hours and give IV frusemide
1 mg/kg at the start of the transfusion. Monitor carefully
for worsening heart failure.**

Try not to transfuse again until at least 4 days have passed.

Intestinal parasites

Routine deworming > 1 year but only in phase 2 or transition
  phase.
Mebendazole 1 tab = 100 mg.

	Single dose	Dose over 3 days
> 1 year of age	500 mg	100 mg twice daily for 3 days

Dermatosis of kwashiokor

- Leave area exposed to dry.
- Apply barrier cream (zinc and castor oil ointment) or
  petroleum jelly or tulle grasse to the raw areas and gentian
  violet or nystatin cream to the skin sores.
- Broad spectrum antibiotics.
- Do not use plastic pants or disposable nappies.
- Give zinc supplements.

Continuing diarrhoea

Giardiasis and mucosal damage are common causes. Where
possible, examine stools by microscopy. If cysts or
trophozoites of *Giardia lamblia* are found, give
metronidazole (5 mg/kg 8 hourly for 7 days).

Diarrhoea is rarely due to lactose intolerance. Only treat for
lactose intolerance if the continuing diarrhoea is preventing
general improvement. Starter F-75 is a low-lactose feed.
In exceptional cases:

- Substitute milk feeds with yoghurt or a lactose-free infant formula.
- Reintroduce milk feeds gradually in the rehabilitation phase.

Osmotic diarrhoea

If diarrhoea worsens substantially with hyperosmolar F-75 and ceases when the sugar content and osmolarity are reduced. In these cases:

- Use a lower osmolar cereal-based starter F-75 or, if available, use a commercially prepared isotonic starter F-75.
- Introduce catch-up F-100 gradually.

Malaria: treatment and prevention

In endemic areas, a rapid malaria smear on admission. Give standard local treatment. Sleep under impregnated nets in the wards.

Tuberculosis

TB can be a cause of failure to gain weight.
Children with TB should not be isolated.

Dietary treatment in phase 1

Principles

Feeding:

- Should start quickly during the admission process.
- Should be divided into many small meals to prevent hypoglycaemia and hypothermia.
- Encourage but not force to eat. Use a cup or a bowl or a spoon or syringe to feed weak children. If takes < 70% of prescribed diet, NG tube.
- Always continue breastfeeding; after breastfeed give scheduled amounts of starter formula.
- Night feeds are essential.
- 100 kcal/kg/day.
- Protein: 1–1·5 g/kg/day.

- Liquid: 130 ml/kg/day (to all children no matter what their state of oedema is).

A recommended schedule is as follows:

Days	Frequency	Vol/kg/feed	Vol/kg/day
1–2	2 hourly	11 ml	130 ml
3–5	3 hourly	16 ml	130 ml
6 onwards	4 hourly	22 ml	130 ml

Special milk for phase 1 is F-75 has: 75 kcal/100 ml:
- 0·9 g of protein/100 ml (around 5% kcal provided by protein)
- 2 g of fat/100 ml (around 32% of kcal provided by fat)
- 13 g of carbohydrate/100 ml (around 62% of kcal provided by carbohydrates)

F-75: 133 ml = 100 kcal.
Do not exceed 100 kcal/kg/day in this initial phase.

Home made phase 1 diet
Note: commercial F-75 starter mix is much better than home made because contains maltodextrin instead of sugar and does not have high osmolality of home made preparation, which can cause an osmotic diarrhoea. Alternatively 35 g/L of starch can be added and the sugar reduced to 70 g/L.

Food item	Quantity
Dried skimmed milk (DSM)	25 g
or boiled full cream milk	300 ml
Vegetable oil	27 g (30 ml)
Sugar	105 g
Water (boiled)	Add water to make 1 litre of preparation
CMV*	20 ml (should be added after the water)

* Minerals and vitamin mix.

Acute liver failure

Grades of hepatic encephalopathy

Grade	Symptoms
I	Irritable. Inappropriate behaviour. Difficulty in writing Lethargy. Mildly depressed awareness Tremor or flap (slow wave in outstretched extended hand)
II	Aggressive outbursts. Bad language Unable to stay still Pulling at IV cannulae/plaster, etc. Mood swings
III	Irritable, odd behaviour (can be associated with raised intracranial pressure (RICP)) Not recognising parents (can be associated with RICP) Flapping tremor Photophobia
IV a	Mostly sleeping but rousable (can be associated with RICP) Flapping tremor (can be associated with RICP) Incoherent, sluggish pupils, hypertonia ± Clonus, extensor spasm
IVb	Absent reflexes Irregular gasps with imminent respiratory failure (can be associated with RICP) Bradycardia Unresponsive to painful stimuli

- If encephalopathy, nurse head elevated at 30° in neutral position.
- Sedation worsens encephalopathy: do not give sedation.
- Aim for two-thirds maintenance fluid intake.
- Maintain blood glucose between 4 and 9 mmol/L using minimal fluid volume, typically 40–60 ml/kg/day of crystalloid (0·9% saline or Hartmann's) with high glucose concentrations, for example 10% (100 g/L – add 200 ml of 50% glucose to a litre of 0·9% saline) or 20% (200 g/litre – add 400 ml of 50% glucose to a litre of 0·9% saline). The 20% solution is irritant to peripheral veins and is best given orally or via NG tube or, if not tolerated, into a central vein.

- Hypoxaemia prevented with O_2 by nasal cannulae or facemask.
- Strict monitoring of urinary output and fluid balance. Aim for urine output of not < 0·5 ml/kg/h (determined by weighing nappies or measuring output). Allow for hot climate and 10% extra fluid for each degree of fever.
- Daily weights.
- If possible insert central venous line and aim for CVP of 6–10 cm H_2O. Increased CVP may be required to compensate for an increased cardiac output or to treat reduced cardiac performance seen as liver failure progresses.
- Manage hypotension with IV colloids and possibly dopamine and epinephrine infusions.
- Inotropes for cardiogenic shock.
- Give no potassium whilst anuric. Metabolic alkalosis may cause hypokalaemia which worsens encephalopathy – correct enterally or IV.
- Stop oral protein initially and during recovery gradually reintroduce 0·5–1 g/kg/day oral or NG.
- A high energy intake, predominantly of dietary carbohydrate.
- Lactulose 5–10 ml 2–3/day to produce between two and four soft and acid stools per day (omit if diarrhoea).
- Maintain normo-thermia by environmental measures (NOT with paracetamol).
- Give 1 dose of IV or IM vitamin K (300 micrograms/kg aged 1 month to 12 years: 10 mg for > 12 years).
- If bleeding (GIT or other) fresh frozen plasma or cryoprecipitate at 10 ml/kg IV.
- Prophylactic H_2 blocking agent (for example, ranitidine 2 mg/kg twice daily IV plus oral antacid (for example, sucralfate 250 mg four times a day 1 month to 2 years, 500 mg four times a day 2–12 years, 1 g four times a day 12–18 years) to prevent gastric/duodenal ulceration.
- Broad spectrum antibiotics, for example, a cephalosporin plus amoxicillin *or* penicillin plus gentamicin. Treat any confirmed sepsis aggressively.

- Systemic fungal infection may require IV amphoterin B (250 micrograms to 1 mg/kg/day) or oral fluconazole (5 mg/kg × 2/day).
- Prophylactic oral nystatin mouthwashes (100 000 IU (1 ml) × 4/day).
- N-acetylcysteine 100 mg/kg/day as continuous infusion in all forms of liver failure.

If **paracetamol overdose** is suspected or ascertained, (see p 42), N-acetylcysteine immediately, whatever time since overdose. 150 mg/kg over 15 minutes as a loading dose then 100 mg/kg over 12 hours then 100 mg/kg/day as a continuous infusion until international normalised ratio (INR) is normal.

Acute renal failure (ARF)

Prerenal (shock induced)

If fractional excretion of sodium (FENa) < 1%, renal tubules alive and responding to shock by reabsorbing sodium. (see Appendix, p 188)

Treatment

- Give 10–20 ml/kg 0·9% saline or colloid as rapidly as possible, and repeat if necessary.
- Then 0·9% saline to fully correct the fluid deficit within 2–4 hours. The deficit in ml = child's weight × % dehydration × 10 (for example, a 6 kg infant 10% dehydrated is deficient of 600 ml). Would receive between 60 and 240 ml of colloid very rapidly, and the rest of the 600 ml as 0·9% saline.
- Once rehydration begun, frusemide 2 mg/kg orally or IV.
- If shock remains after rehydration, it may be cardiogenic; consider inotropes.

Established ARF

FENa > 2%. Trial of frusemide 2 mg/kg orally IV.

Management of persistent ARF

Meticulous fluid balance measuring all intakes and losses, especially if oliguric (< 1 ml/kg/h). Insensible water loss = 300 ml/m^2 (12 ml/kg/24h in > 1 year and 15 ml/kg/24 hr in infancy) in temperate conditions, and higher in hotter climates, at low humidity and with fever.

Weigh twice daily.

Nutrition, fluid and electrolyte balance:

- Difficult in oligo-anuric ARF. Solid food is best. Provide calories from carbohydrates and fats, and limit protein to 1 g/kg/day.
- Limit salt intake to prevent sodium retention and hypernatraemia (leads to insatiable thirst) and fluid overload.
- Provide some sodium as bicarbonate to prevent acidosis = 1 mmol/kg/day (1 ml of 8·4% sodium bicarbonate solution = 1 mmol, and 1 g of powder = 12 mmol).
- Dietary potassium must be restricted.
- Dietary phosphate restricted by giving calcium carbonate with the food (for example, 0·5–2 grams with each meal). Also prevents hypocalcaemia.

Dialysis for prolonged oligo-anuria, hyperkalaemia, severe metabolic acidosis due to difficulty of giving bicarbonate, hypoglycaemia, clinical uraemia (> 40 mmol/L), and need for other fluids such as platelets.

Hyperkalaemia

Causes arrhythmias, especially in ARF where other metabolic changes such as hypocalcaemia. Keep K below 6·5 mmol/L in older child and below 7·0 mmol/L in neonates.

- Reduce effects on heart by increasing plasma Ca. Give 0·5 ml/kg (0·1 mmol/kg) of 10% calcium gluconate.
- Remove K$^+$ from body by calcium resonium 1 g/kg orally or rectally, and repeat 0·5 g/kg 12 hourly.
- Push K$^+$ into cells. Lasts only a few hours:

- Using salbutamol. Nebulise 2·5 mg for children under 25 kg, and 5 mg in larger children, or give 5 micrograms/kg IV over 5 minutes.
- Infuse a high concentration of glucose (5 ml/kg 10% glucose over 20 minutes). Monitor plasma glucose and infuse insulin at 0·05 units/kg/h if it exceeds 12 mmol/L. It is unsafe to mix the glucose and insulin and infuse together as may cause hypoglycaemia.
- Give 2·5 mmol/kg of NaHCO$_3$ over 15 minutes. If 8·4% is used, containing 1 mmol/ml, will increase plasma Na by approximately 5 mmol/L very quickly. Better to use a solution of 1·26% which is isonatraemic, but requires 17 ml/kg to be infused, adding to fluid overload.

Neurological

Bacterial meningitis

- **Older child:** fever, neck stiffness, vomiting, headache, altered consciousness, and possibly seizures.
- **Neonates:** signs more subtle and non-specific and include poor feeding, hyper- or hypothermia, convulsions, apnoea, irritability, and a bulging fontanelle.
- Contraindications to lumbar puncture are raised intracranial pressure, too sick to tolerate flexed position, infection at puncture site, bleeding tendency, or rash suggesting meningococcal disease. Antibiotics started and lumbar puncture delayed until safe.
- In malarial areas undertake blood smear and treat if suspicion.
- Consider TB meningitis if no response to initial antibiotics and if two or more present from:
  - History > 7 days
  - HIV known or suspected
  - Patient remains unconscious
  - CSF continues to have high WBC count (typically $< 500 \times 10^9/l$ mostly lymphocytes, elevated protein ($0\cdot8$–4 g/L), and low glucose ($< 1\cdot5$ mmol/L)
  - CXR suggesting TB, optic atrophy, focal neurological deficit, or extrapyramidal movements.
- HIV prone to meningitis and septicaemia from *Streptococcus pneumoniae* and salmonella.
- *Listeria monocytogenes* headache but little neck stiffness.
- Fungal infections in HIV, severe headache without neck stiffness.
- Antibiotic choice depends on known local effectiveness, CSF penetration, cost and availability, and local patterns of antibiotic resistance. Treat according to age group.

Third generation cephalosporins drugs of choice for *Haemophilus influenzae* and meningococcus organisms although, if precluded on cost, chloramphenicol acceptable alternative. Pneumococci resistant to penicillin and to chloramphenicol are widespread, and third generation cephalosporins are then drugs of choice. However, pneumococcal resistance to third generation cephalosporins is found requiring addition of vancomycin or rifampicin to third generation cephalosporins. In neonates ceftazidime which is active against pseudomonas is useful.

- Give antibiotics in neonates 14–21 days; children 10 days for pneumococcal and haemophilus, 7 days for meningococcal infections.
- Dexamethasone 150 micrograms/kg 6 hourly for 2 days. First dose with or max. 4 hours after first antibiotic dose.
- In TB meningitis dexamethasone 150 micrograms/kg 6 hourly for 2–3 weeks, tailing down the dose over a further 2–3 weeks.
- Do not use steroids in: the newborn, suspected cerebral malaria, or viral encephalitis.

Typical findings in CSF

See table on page 100.

Supportive care

- **Fluids:** correct shock or dehydration initially IV later by NG tube or orally. Avoid overhydration by careful fluid balance and in particular avoid IV fluids with low sodium levels such as 5% dextrose. Use 0·9% saline plus 10% glucose. Maintain serum Na$^+$ high normal range > 135 mmol/L. NG tube if unconscious or vomiting to protect airway. Milk (1 ml/kg/h) to prevent gastric erosions and improve bowel function. Urine output monitored, particularly if unconscious.

Condition	White cell count (× 10^9/L)	Cell differential	Protein (g/L)	Glucose (mmol/L)
Normal	0–5 <22 in full term, <30 in preterm	PMN ≤ 2 <15 neonate	<0·5	2/3 blood glucose
Acute bacterial meningitis*	100 – >300 000	Mostly PMN Monocytes in *Listeria* sp.	>1·0	<2·5
Tuberculosis meningitis	50–500 sometimes higher	Lymphocytes but PMN early	>1·0	<2·5, usually 0
Herpes encephalitis	Usually < 500	Mostly lymphocytes PMN early in the disease	>0·5	Normal
Cerebral abscess	10–200	PMN or lymphocytes	>1·0	Normal
Traumatic tap	WBC and RBC	RBC/WBC = 500/1	↑ by 0·001 g/L per 1000 RBC	Normal

*Bacterial meningitis can occur without pleocytosis and partial treatment will alter findings.
PMN = polymorphonuclear granulocytes

- **Seizures:** controlled with anticonvulsants, but not prophylactic.
- **Temperature control:** if high fever (> 38°C) apply temperature reduction including paracetamol.
- **Glucose control:** regularly monitored particularly infant and young child. Hypoglycaemia considered in seizures or altered consciousness and corrected as follows: 5 ml/kg of 10% glucose IV and recheck blood glucose 30 minutes later. If remains low (< 2·5 mmol/L) repeat.
- **Nutritional support:** NG if unable to feed after 48 h. Continue expressed breastmilk or give milk feeds 15 ml/kg every 3 hours.
- Turn unconscious child 2 hourly, keeping dry, and prevent overheating.

Antibiotic therapy: depends on local resistance, national guidelines and availability

Give all IV for at least 72 hours or longer if unwell or fever continues.

See table on page 102.

Organism	Antibiotics of choice	Alternative antibiotics	Duration
Haemophilus influenzae	Ceftriaxone or cefotaxime	Chloramphenicol plus ampicillin	10–14 days
Streptococcus pneumoniae	Ceftriaxone or cefotaxime	Chloramphenicol plus benzyl penicillin	10–14 days
Neisseria meningitidis	Ceftriaxone or cefotaxime	Chloramphenicol plus benzyl penicillin	7 days
Gram negative bacilli	Gentamicin plus ampicillin or ceftriaxone/cefotaxime	Chloramphenicol plus ampicillin or ceftazidime	At least 21 days, repeat LP to ensure CSF response
Salmonella enteritides	As for gram negative bacilli plus IV ciprofloxacin	Meropenem or chloramphenicol plus ampicillin	At least 21 days, repeat LP to ensure CSF response
Listeria monocytogenes	Ampicillin plus gentamicin		10–14 days
Group B streptococcus	Benzylpenicillin plus gentamicin or ceftriaxone or cefotaxime		10–14 days
Staphylococcus spp.	Gentamicin and flucloxacillin	Chloramphenicol* plus flucloxacillin	10–14 days

* Chloramphenicol with caution < 3 months – monitor levels.

Antibiotic	Route	Dose
Ampicillin	IV	100 mg/kg 6 hourly (max single dose 3 g)
Benzylpenicillin	IV	50 mg/kg 4 hourly
Cefotaxime	IV	50 mg/kg 4 hourly (max single dose 4 g)
Ceftriaxone	IV/IM	80 mg/kg 24hours once daily* (max single dose 4 g)
Chloramphenicol	IV	25 mg/kg 6 hourly (after loading dose of 50 mg/kg)
	Oral	25 mg/kg 6 hourly†
	IM	Only prep. in doses of 50–100 mg/kg 12 hourly with a max dose of 3 g
Ciprofloxacin	IV	10 mg/kg 12 hourly (5 mg/kg 12 hourly in neonate)
Flucloxacillin or cloxacillin	IV	50 mg/kg 6 hourly (max. dose 8 g/day)
Gentamicin	IV or IM	1 month to 12 years 6 mg/kg once daily, † > 12 yrs 4–5 mg/kg once daily
Meropenem	IV	40 mg/kg 8 hourly (max. single dose 2 g) slow IV over 5 min (>12 years 600 mg once daily)
Vancomycin	IV	15 mg/kg loading dose and then 10 mg/kg 6 hourly‡

* Ideally 80 mg/kg 12 hourly should be given for the first 3 doses followed by 80 mg/kg per 24 hours.
† Not recommended in children less than 3 months old or in malnourished children
‡ Monitoring levels important

Endocrine and metabolic

Diabetic ketoacidosis (DKA)

Suspect if:
- Dehydration:
- Abdominal pain
- Ketone smell on breath
- Acidosis with acidotic breathing
- Unexplained coma.

In DKA death is from hypokalaemia or cerebral oedema.
Cerebral oedema is unpredictable, and is more frequent in
young and new diabetics.

Emergency management of children > 5% dehydrated and clinically unwell

1. **General resuscitation:**
    ABCD.

2. **Confirm diagnosis:**
    History : polydipsia, polyuria
    Clinical : acidotic respiration; dehydration; drowsiness;
    abdominal pain/vomiting
    Biochemical : high blood glucose on finger-prick; ketones
    or glucose in urine.

3. **Investigations:**
    Weigh or estimate from centile charts (then twice daily)
    Blood glucose
    Urea and electrolytes and blood gas
    PCV and full blood count
    Blood culture
    Urine microscopy, culture and sensitivity
    ECG to observe T waves (hypokalaemia = flat T waves;
    hyperkalaemia = peaked T waves).

Other investigations if indicated, for example chest x ray, CSF, throat swab, etc. (DKA may be precipitated by sepsis, and **fever is not part of DKA**.)

Assess and record

1. **Degree of dehydration:**
   < 5%: dry mucous membranes
   6–9%: as above plus sunken eyes and reduced skin turgor, plus restless and irritable
   ≥ 10%: as above plus shock: severely ill with poor perfusion (capillary return > 2 sec) thready rapid pulse, reduced blood pressure, rapid deep breathing, altered consciousness or coma.
   Strict fluid balance essential.

2. **Conscious level:**
   Assess AVPU (**A**lert; responds to **V**oice; responds to **P**ain; **U**nresponsive)
   Institute hourly neurological observations. If less than **A**lert on admission, or deterioration, record Glasgow Coma Score and transfer to ICU. Consider cerebral oedema management.
   Cerebral oedema – irritability, headache, (late signs = slow **pulse, high blood pressure,** and papilloedema).

Management

1. **Fluids:**
   If shocked, resuscitate by restoring circulatory volume with bolus of 20 ml/kg 0·9% saline.
   It is rare to need > one 20 ml/kg fluid bolus for resuscitation – too much fluid too quickly can cause cerebral oedema.

$$\text{Requirement} = \text{Maintenance} + \text{Deficit}$$
$$\text{Deficit (in ml)} = \% \text{ dehydration} \times \text{body weight (kg)} \times 10$$

Avoid overzealous fluid replacement, which risks cerebral oedema. **Calculate deficit to a maximum of 8% dehydration**. *Ignore fluids given to resuscitate.*

Add maintenance and deficit and give total evenly over 24 hours.

Glucose > 12 mmol/L – give 0·9% saline

Glucose < 12 mmol/L – give 0·45% saline + 5% dextrose

Sodium 135–155 correct over 24 hours

Sodium > 155 correct over 48 hours using no lower concentration than 0·45% saline

Expect the sodium to rise initially as glucose falls and water is removed from circulation*

*To prevent cerebral oedema, if Na is falling, change from 0·45% to 0·9% saline.

2. **Bicarbonate:**
   Rarely, if ever, necessary. Only if profoundly acidotic (pH < 7·0) and shocked with circulatory failure, to improve cardiac contractility. **Half-correct** acidosis over 60 minutes:

   Volume (ml 4·2% $NaHCO_3$) = 1/3 × body weight (kg) × base deficit (mmol/L) = half-correction.

3. **Potassium:**
   Give immediately unless anuria, peaked T waves on ECG or K^+ > 7·0 mmol/L.
   Always massive depletion of total body potassium although initial plasma levels may be low, normal, or even high. Levels will fall once insulin is commenced.
   Add 20 mmol KCl to every 500 ml unit of fluid given.
   Check urea and electrolytes (U&E's) 2 hours after resuscitation, then 4 hourly, alter K^+ input accordingly.
   Observe ECG frequently.

4. **Insulin:**
   Continuous low dose IV is the preferred method. No initial bolus.

Make 1 unit per ml of human soluble insulin (for example, Actrapid) by adding 50 units (0·5 ml) insulin to 50 ml 0·9% saline. Attach using a Y-connector to IV fluids already running.* Do not add insulin directly to fluid bags. Solution should then run at 0·1 units/kg/h (0·1 ml/kg/h).

If rate of blood glucose fall exceeds 5 mmol/L per hour, reduce insulin infusion rate to 0·05 units/kg/h.
Once blood glucose is < 12 mmol/L, and glucose-containing fluid started, consider reducing insulin infusion rate.
Do not stop insulin infusion while glucose infused.
If blood glucose < 7 mmol/L, consider adding extra glucose to infusion.
If blood glucose rises re-evaluate (? sepsis or other condition), and consider re-starting protocol.

If no syringe pump, give SC boluses of actrapid 6 hourly at 0·6 units/kg/dose (that is 0·1 units/kg/h). Give half dose if the blood sugar falling too fast.

Cerebral oedema in DKA

Signs and symptoms

Headache	Confusion
Irritability	Reduced conscious level
Fits	Small pupils
Increasing BP, slowing pulse	Possibly respiratory impairment

Management

- Exclude hypoglycaemia.
- Give mannitol 250–500 mg/kg (1·25–2·5 ml/kg mannitol 20%) over 15 minutes as soon as suspected.
- **Restrict IV fluids to two-third maintenance.**

- Intubate and ventilate; keep $PaCO_2$ to 3·5–5·0 kPa. **Keep Na > 135 mmol/L. Keep head in midline and 30 degrees elevated. Avoid fever > 38·0° C.**
- Repeat mannitol every 4–6 hours to control ICP.

Adrenal crisis

Diagnosis

- Most in neonates with congenital adrenal hyperplasia (CAH) or hypopituitarism (**virilisation in the female** with CAH and **micropenis and cryptorchidism** in male with hypopituitarism).
- Those receiving long term steroid therapy or adrenal destruction secondary to **autoimmune process or tuberculosis**.
- Suspect in severely ill with:

  - Acidosis
  - Hyponatraemia
  - Hypotension
  - Hyperkalaemia
  - Hypoglycaemia
  - And in child receiving long term steroid therapy

Replacement hydrocortisone up to 15 mg/m²/day replicates natural secretion. Therapy with hydrocortisone > 15 mg/m²/day produces suppression related to dose and duration. (1 mg prednisolone = approx. 3 mg hydrocortisone).

In patients on steroids, for emergency stress, the dose of oral is usually three times replacement dose. If given parenterally as treatment for operative cover or illness associated with vomiting = hydrocortisone (12·5 mg for infants, 25 mg for children, 50 mg for older children, and 100 mg for adults given 4–6 hourly IV or IM).

Management

- ABCD and treat hypoglycaemia.
- Continue 0·9% saline to correct deficit and for maintenance.
- Give hydrocortisone IV 4 hourly as follows: dose: 12·5 mg for neonate and infant; 25 mg for 1–5 years, 50 mg for 6–12 years, and 100 mg for 13–18 years.
- If diagnosis established, continue maintenance hydrocortisone 15 mg/m^2 per day in 3 divided doses and, if salt loss demonstrated, fludrocortisone 150–250 micrograms/m^2/day once daily with sodium chloride 1G/10 kg/day (60 mg = 1 mmol).

Hypoglycaemia

Treatment of hypoglycaemia

- Symptoms non-specific, always consider blood glucose.
- Treat any ill child with suspicious symptoms: fits, encephalopathy, or condition associated with hypoglycaemia, such as severe malnutrition or malaria.
- Give glucose orally if safe (0·5–1·0 g/kg). If conscious and able to eat, give food or sugary fluids.
- Otherwise 2–5 ml/kg 10% dextrose IV over 3 minutes. **Never use stronger glucose solutions.** Continue with 0·1 ml/kg/min 10% dextrose to maintain blood sugar 5–8 mmol/L.
- If hypoadrenalism/pituitarism is suspected give hydrocortisone (see above).
- If IV access lost give glucagon IM 20 micrograms/kg (max. 1 mg as single dose) (especially if on insulin).

Hypokalaemia

Treatment of severe hypokalaemia

High potassium IV infusions.

Maximum concentration IV 4 mmol/100 ml (either 5% glucose or 0.9% saline)

At a rate of not exceeding 0.5 mmol/kg/h ideally with ECG monitoring

If acidotic, bicarbonate should only be given if serum K >3 mmol/L

Watch serum magnesium levels if possible

A urine K^+ > 25 mmol/L confirms renal potassium loss

Infectious diseases

Diphtheria

- Admit to isolation to be cared for by immunised staff.
- Protect airway if possible by intubation/tracheostomy.
- **Dexamethasone (0·6 mg/kg 12 hourly IV or oral) for airway obstruction and neck swelling.**
- Benzylpenicillin 50 mg/kg 4 hourly IV or erythromycin 10 mg/kg 6 hourly (max. 2 g/day) IV.

Antitoxin

Administer immediately after test dose, dependent on severity:

nasal and tonsillar (mild disease) 20 000 units IM
laryngeal with symptoms (moderately severe)
   40 000 units IM/IV
nasopharyngeal (moderately severe) 60–100 000 units IV
combined sites/delayed diagnosis (malignant disease)
   60–100 000 units IV.

In practice 60 000 units to all with visible membrane and neck swelling.

Antitoxin is *horse serum*: test dose 0·1 ml of 1 in 1000 dilution in saline given intradermally.
Positive reaction is 10 mm erythema occurring within 20 minutes.
If no reaction, give full dose IV/IM as appropriate.
Have epinephrine 1 in 1000 available to give IM if anaphylaxis (10 micrograms/kg).

Desensitisation

Give graduated doses of increased strength every 20 minutes commencing with: 0·1 ml of 1 in 20 dilution in saline SC followed by 1 in 10 dilution, 0·1 ml of undiluted SC then 0·3 ml and 0·5 ml IM. Then 0·1 ml undiluted IV.

- O_2 if cyanosed or $SaO_2 < 94\%$. Use nasal cannulae or facemask held close to child's face by the mother. DO NOT use nasopharyngeal catheters as can precipitate complete airway obstruction. Be aware O_2 does NOT compensate for hypoventilation which if severe will require intubation or surgical airway. Laryngoscopy may dislodge membrane producing complete airway obstruction.

Bed rest and observation

- Monitor cardiac function for 2–3 weeks.
- Serial ECGs for arrhythmias – pacemaker may be needed.
- For cardiac failure give captopril 100 micrograms/kg as test dose supine and monitor BP carefully then 100–200 micrograms/kg 8 hourly.
- Prednisolone 1·5 mg/kg/day for 2 weeks may reduce incidence of myocarditis.
- NG feeds if palatal or bulbar paralysis.

Meningococcal disease

- Give IV/IM benzylpenicillin before transfer to hospital:

  < 1 year = 300 mg
  1–10 years = 600 mg
  > 10 years = 1·2g.

- On admission benzylpenicillin plus cefotaxime IV are most appropriate antibiotics (see Table for doses and other antibiotics).
- Treat shock and raised intracranial pressure (see pages 22 and 31).
- Treat any coagulopathy with vitamin K, FFP, cryoprecipitate and platelets as required.
- Do not undertake LP.
- Prophylaxis to contacts.

Dengue haemorrhagic shock

Treat shock and other effects (such as bleeding disorder) as for meningococcal septicaemia.

Antibiotic doses in meningococcal disease

Antibiotic	Route	Dose
Benzylpenicillin	IV	300 mg/kg 24 h in 6 divided doses
Cefotaxime	IV	200 mg/kg 24 h in 4 divided doses (max. single dose 4 g)
Ceftriaxone*	IV/IM	80 mg/kg 24 h once daily* (max. single dose 4 g)
Chloramphenicol	IV	100 mg/kg 24 h in 4 divided doses†
	Oral	100 mg/kg 24 h in 4 divided doses‡
	IM	IM preparation of oily chloramphenicol in single dose of 50–100 mg/kg with a maximum dose of 3 g; only if more suitable alternatives are unavailable

* Ideally 12 hourly for first 3 doses.
† Chloramphenicol with caution in infants < 3 months.
‡ Oral only after 72 hours of IV/IM.

Tetanus

- Secure and maintain **airway. Ensure adequacy of ventilation.**
- Pharyngeal spasms/upper airway obstruction best managed with a tracheostomy.
- Intubation difficult because of pharyngeal/laryngeal spasm and often a mini-tracheostomy without prior intubation may be appropriate, providing experts on the procedure and on anaesthesia are present.
- Benzylpenicillin 50 mg/kg every 6 hours IV or, if not possible, IM for 48 hours and then oral penicillin 12·5 mg/kg 6 hourly for 7 days. Metronidazole may be useful.
- Anti-tetanus human immunoglobulin **5000–10 000 units immediately** by IV infusion over 30 minutes.
- Alternative equine immunoglobulin 500–1000 units/kg IM (max. dose 20 000 units): risk of anaphylaxis (epinephrine 10 micrograms/kg immediately available).
- If in acute spasm, **diazepam by bolus IV infusion over 15 minutes (dose 200 micrograms/kg) or rectally (500 micrograms/kg).** Ensure IV diazepam is diluted to 100 micrograms/ml and that extravasation does not occur. Give every 3–6 hours or continuous infusion of midazolam (30–100 micrograms/kg/h). But doses needed to control spasms almost invariably cause some degree of respiratory depression so patient MUST be observed continuously.
- If this is not possible, NG diazepam 250–500 micrograms/kg 6 hourly alternating with chlorpromazine 500 micrograms/kg 6 hourly. The first dose of chlorpromazine can be given as a bolus IM if spasms are severe.
- Alternative treatments for spasms:
    baclofen for children > 1 year (start at 750 micrograms/kg/day and increase to 2 mg/kg/day in 3 divided doses)
    phenobarbitone (15 mg/kg in 1 or 2 divided doses as a loading dose and then 5 mg/kg/day)
    paraldehyde (0·4 ml/kg rectally in olive oil or 0·9% saline repeated 4–6 hourly).

- Paracetamol 25 mg/kg 6 hourly for pain (20 mg/kg in the neonate). If this is insufficient the WHO pain ladder approach should be adopted (see page 176). Oral or IV morphine (100 micrograms/kg or 50 micrograms/kg in neonates as loading dose may be needed).
- NG fluids, food and drugs with **minimal disturbance.** Feeds need to be given frequently (ideally hourly) in small amounts due to reduced gut motility.
- Any **wound debrided** and **cleaned** and ill-advised sutures removed.
- In severe cases mechanical ventilation. **Infusions morphine and midazolam, alongside muscle relaxants, minimise suffering.**
- **Good nursing** and **frequent monitoring** with particular attention to **suction of secretions** from the airway, maintenance of adequate **hydration, mouth hygiene,** turning to avoid orthostatic pneumonia and bed sores, will reduce complications.
- Keep mother with child all the time.
- Quiet environment with low level lighting. Sudden loud noises avoided. Invasive procedures minimum and preceded by appropriate analgesia/sedation. **Must be CONTINUOUS observation by experienced personnel.**
- Monitor **ECG** to detect **toxin-induced arrhythmias** and autonomic instability. If present sedate with morphine.
- Associated septicaemia common in neonates (broad spectrum antibiotics will be needed as well as treatment for tetanus).

Typhoid fever

Diagnosis is clinical.

Suspect if high grade fever for > 72 hours with anorexia, vomiting, hepatosplenomegaly, diarrhoea, toxicity, abdominal pain, and pallor *especially with no localising upper respiratory signs or meningitis or malaria*. Leucopenia

(WCC $< 4 \times 10^9$/L) with left shift; but in a third of infants leucocytosis.

Treatment

Early diagnosis.

- Soft, easily digestible diet continued unless abdominal distension or ileus when clear fluids only.
- If no drug resistance in region start with oral chloramphenicol and/or oral amoxicillin/ampicillin (initially IV if vomiting). If drug resistance use cefotaxime, ceftriaxone, or ciprofloxacin.
- If poor response after 72 hours, imipenem.
- In severely ill and toxic, dexamethasone IV (200 micrograms 8 hourly 6 doses).

Drug	Route	Dose (frequency)	Duration (days)
Chloramphenicol	Oral	60–75 mg/kg/24 hours q 6 hourly	14 days
Ampicillin/amoxicillin	IV/oral	100 mg/kg/24 hours q 6–8 hourly	14 days
Ciprofloxacin	Oral/IV	20 mg/kg/24 hours q 12 hourly	7–10 days
Ceftriaxone	IV/IM	65 mg/kg/24 hours once daily	7–14 days
Cefixime	Oral	15 mg/kg/24 hours q 12 hourly	14 days
Imipenem	IV	60 mg/kg/24 hours q 8 hourly	10–14 days

Measles

Clinical features

- Prodromal priod (3–5 days): acute coryza with fever, cough, and conjunctivitis. Febrile seizures may occur.
- Koplik's spots by second to fourth day.
- Maculopapular rash (fourth day), on face and neck, behind ears and along hairline and becomes generalised after 3 days. Fades after 5–6 days in order of appearance, developing brownish colour and often scaly. If severe petechiae and ecchymoses.
- Fever after third day of rash = complications.

HIV infection with limited access to laboratory in endemic area

Specific to HIV	Uncommon in HIV negative	Common in HIV positive and ill non HIV infected
Pneumocystis pneumonia	Molluscum contagiosum with multiple lesions	Persistent diarrhoea (> 14 days)
Oesophageal candidiasis	Oral thrush (especially after the neonatal period, without antibiotic, > 1 month or recurrent)	Failure to thrive (especially in breastfed infants)
Herpes zoster		Persistent cough (> 1 month)
Lymphoid interstitial pneumonia	Generalised pruritic dermatitis	Generalised lymphadenopathy
Kaposi's sarcoma	Recurrent severe infections (three or more in 1 year)	Hepatosplenomegaly
Chronic parotid enlargement	Persistent and/or recurrent fever lasting > 1 week	
	Neurological dysfunction (progressive neurological impairment)	

Clinical features of severe measles

Signs	Complications
Cough, tachypnoea, or chest indrawing	Pneumonia
Stridor when quiet	Croup, necrotising tracheitis
Severe diarrhoea	Dehydration
Recent severe weight loss	Malnutrition
Corneal damage or Bitot spots	Blindness
Ear discharge	Otitis media, deafness
Lethargy, convulsions	Encephalitis
Inability to drink or eat	Dehydration, malnutrition
Blood in the stools	Dysentery, haemorrhagic measles
Severe stomatitis	Cancrum oris

Management

- Vitamin A capsule 200 000 IU (> 1 year) or 100 000 IU (< 1 year). **Give second dose after 24 hours.**
- Oral hygiene; 1% gentian violet to mouth sores. Treat oral thrush.
- If mouth ulcers infected, use antibiotic (penicillin or metronidazole) orally for 5 days.
- If mouth too sore to feed or drink, NG tube.
- Ocular hygiene for purulent conjunctivitis, daily washings (with sterile 0·9% saline or boiled water using cotton wool swabs and tetracycline eye ointment 3 times daily). NEVER USE TOPICAL STEROIDS. Consider protective eye pads.
- Oral rehydration solution for diarrhoea; ReSoMal if severe malnutrition.
- Antibiotic, oxygen if pneumonia.
- Rapidly spreading pulmonary tuberculosis may occur.
- Croup (see page 67).
- Otitis media. Antibiotics and regular aural hygiene. Screen for hearing impairment during follow-up.
- Xerophthalmia – protective eye pad, give vitamin A capsules (see above).
- Malnutrition (see pages 79–92).
- Encephalopathy (see pages 31–34).

Rabies

Risk of exposure to rabies

- Is bite with broken skin? Have mucous membranes or existing skin lesion been contaminated?
- How did the animal behave? An unprovoked attack by frantic or paralysed dog or unusually tame wild mammal high risk.
- Is biting animal a local rabies vector, or could it have been infected?
- If possible have the animal's brain examined for rabies. Alternatively animal kept under safe observation, and stop vaccine treatment if healthy after 10 days.

Post-exposure treatment (very urgent)

1. **Wound care**

   Scrub and flush lesion with **soap or detergent and water.** Remove foreign material. Local analgesia may be necessary.

   Apply povidone iodine (or 70% ethyl alcohol, but is painful).

   Do not suture wound; delay it.

   Tetanus immunisation.

   Treat bacterial infection of wounds with oral antibiotic.

2. **Rabies vaccine: three post-exposure regimens**

A. **Standard IM regimen**

   One ampoule (1 ml or 0·5 ml) IM into the deltoid, or anterolateral thigh in small children, on days 0, 3, 7, 14, and 28, a total of 5 doses. Do not inject into the buttock.

B. **Economical eight-site intradermal (ID) regimen**

   (Use vaccines containing 1 ml per ampoule. Total of less than 2 ampoules needed.)

   Day 0: draw up 1 ml of vaccine into 1 ml (Mantoux type) syringe. Inject 0·1 ml ID into each of eight sites

(deltoid, thigh, suprascapular and lower anterior
abdominal wall) using all the vaccine.
Day 7 give 0·1 ml ID into four sites (deltoid and
thighs).
Days 28 and 90, 0·1 ml ID at one site.

(This regimen is the treatment of choice when RIG is not
available.)

C. **Economical two-site ID regimen**
Dose: 0·1 ml for purified vero cell vaccine (PVRV) and
0·2 ml for all other vaccines.
Days 0, 3 and 7, give ID into two sites (deltoids).
Days 28 and 90, ID dose at one site.

Regimens B and C: Take care that ID injections raise
a papule. If vaccine subcutaneous, repeat injection
nearby.

If **treatment delayed** > 48 hours after bite, or
immunosuppression suspected (for example, severely
malnourished, AIDS, or corticosteroids therapy), give the first
dose of an IM course ID at eight sites (see **B** above), or for
two-site regimen **(C)**, double the first dose. No change in
dosage for the eight-site regimen.

3. **Rabies immunoglobulin (RIG)**
Plus vaccine following all contacts with suspected rabid
animals where skin broken or mucous membranes
contaminated.
Vital for bites on head, neck, hands, or multiple bites.
Dosage: equine RIG (40 IU/kg) or human RIG (20 IU/kg)
infiltrated into and around wound on day 0. If not
anatomically possible (for example, on a finger) inject any
remainder IM, at a place remote from vaccine site, but not
into the buttock.
Epinephrine 10 micrograms/kg IM to be available.

Postexposure treatment for previously vaccinated patients

One dose of vaccine IM or ID on days 0 and 3. RIG is not necessary. Treatment and thorough wound care is still **urgent**.

Malaria

Clinical features

- Typical features include high grade fever alternating with cold spells, rigors, chills, and sweating. There are usually associated myalgias and arthralgias.
- < 5 years non-specific with fever, vomiting, diarrhoea, abdominal pain main symptoms.
- In older immune individuals only symptoms may be fever with headache and joint pains.

So all fevers in endemic area due to malaria until proven otherwise.

Diagnosis

Blood smear for malaria; thick slide for diagnosis, thin slide to confirm type of malarial parasite. Typically ring forms inside RBCs are seen but there may also be gametocytes. Level of parasitaemia usually scored as 1–4 + (if ≥ 3 = parasitaemia).

Severe malaria

- Child is febrile and has a positive blood smear.
- As temperature fluctuates, a single reading may be normal.
- Vomiting, diarrhoea, or cough.
- Conscious state altered, history of convulsions.
- Hypoglycaemia and acidosis or severe anaemia, jaundice, or generalised weakness (unable to sit up).

Cerebral malaria

Due to *Plasmodium falciparum*. Altered consciousness, severe anaemia, acidosis, or any combination of these. In endemic areas, commonest cause of coma; especially age 1–5 years.

Coma develops rapidly, within 1–2 days of onset of fever, sometimes within hours. Convulsions are usual and may be repeated. Clinical features suggest a metabolic encephalopathy, with raised intracranial pressure. Opisthotonos, decorticate, or decerebrate posturing, hypotonia, and conjugate eye movements are common. Oculovestibular reflexes and pupillary responses usually intact. Papilloedema in a minority.

Hypoglycaemia, acidosis, hyperpyrexia, and convulsions (sometimes undetectable without EEG) are common.

Other causes of coma, such as meningitis, must be sought, and if necessary treated.

Investigations

Thick and thin films for malarial parasites.
Blood glucose.
Lumbar puncture if meningitis suspected – contraindications
  include: Glasgow Coma Scale < 8, papilloedema or
  suspicion of raised intracranial pressure including a tense
  fontanelle in infants, or respiratory difficulty. In such a
  situation, give IV antibiotics as well as anti-malarials (see
  page 98).

Management of severe malaria

- Treat convulsions (see page 37).
- Treat hypoglycaemia (< 2·5 mmol/L in well nourished;
  < 3·5 mmol/L in malnourished children; see page 86).
- Treat shock and dehydration.
- **Initiate antimalarial therapy** (pages 22 and 75):
  If blood smear not immediately available and no other
  obvious cause treat as malaria. In Africa and many other

regions quinine is drug of choice for severe malaria. In SE Asia and Amazon basin quinine is no longer always effective. Initially give treatment IV, if possible; if not, IM. Change to oral therapy as soon as possible.

First line – quinine IV

- Give 20 mg salt/kg in 20 ml/kg of 5% dextrose over 4–6 hours. Use an in-line infusion chamber (100–150 ml) to ensure that the loading dose does not go in too quickly. There is a major risk of cardiac side effects if this happens. If safe control over rate of infusion of IV quinine not possible, give IM (10 mg/kg load and then 10 mg/kg at 4 hours).
- Then 10 mg/kg in 10 ml/kg fluid every 12 hours for 24 hours or longer if child remains unconscious. These latter doses can be given over 2 hours.
- Never give bolus infusion.
- As soon as able to take orally, switch to quinine tablets 10 mg/kg every 8 hours for 7 days.
- For IM injections, dilute quinine solution for better absorption and less pain.

Side effects:

Common: cinchonism (tinnitus, hearing loss, nausea and vomiting, uneasiness, restlessness, dizziness, blurring of vision).

Uncommon: hypoglycaemia, although a common complication of severe malaria.

Serious cardiovascular problems (QT prolongation) and neurological toxicity are rare.

If overdosed by mistake with quinine tablets: give activated charcoal orally or by NG tube as a suspension in water (DOSE = 1 g/kg).

Second line antimalarials

Second line drugs include pyrimethamine with sulfadoxine (Fansidar), amiodaquine, metakelfin, and halofantrine. Artemether and mefloquine are currently designated as reserve drugs for multidrug resistant malaria.

Always check local guidelines on drug sensitivities

- Prevent hypoglycaemia with a 10% glucose infusion IV (add 10 ml 50% glucose to 90 ml of 5% glucose solution).
- Treat hypoglycaemia with 5 ml/kg of 10% glucose solution IV. Recheck blood glucose after 30 minutes and repeat glucose bolus if blood glucose is still low. If no IV access, give via NG.
- Treat severe anaemia: blood transfusion if Hb < 5 g/dl or Hct < 15% or evidence of cardiac failure OR if Hb > 5 g/dl (Hct > 15%) but very heavy parasitaemia and falling Hb.
- Give packed cells 10 ml/kg or fresh whole blood 20 ml/kg over 3–4 hours. If severely malnourished, circulatory overload is more likely and give packed cells if possible or partial exchange transfusion (see page 89), if not give IV frusemide (1–2 mg/kg) with 10 ml/kg of whole blood. Diuretics are not normally needed unless there is evidence of fluid overload.
- If unable to swallow NG feeds. When a gag reflex is present introduce oral fluids.
- Nurse in recovery position and turn 2 hourly. Do not allow child to lie in a wet bed and provide special care to pressure points.
- Check blood glucose 4–6 hourly and Hb/Hct daily.
- Watch urine output – aim at 1 ml/kg/h. If despite rehydration urine output is < 4 ml/kg/24 h give IV frusemide 2 mg/kg. If no response double dose at hourly intervals to a maximum of 8 mg/kg.
- Monitor coma score 4 hourly.
- Treat convulsions, hypoglycaemia, hyperpyrexia (> 39°C).
- Shock is unusual in malaria. If present treat with IV boluses of colloid/crystalloid 20 ml/kg and consider septicaemia. Take blood cultures, and start broad spectrum antibiotics IV (penicillin and chloramphenicol OR cefotaxime or ceftriaxone) in addition to antimalarials.

- If there is deep or laboured breathing suggestive of acidosis, give extra IV fluid to correct hypovolaemia.
- During rehydration examine frequently for fluid overload (increased liver, gallop rhythm, fine crackles at lung bases, distended jugular venous pressure).
- Always in infants use an in-line infusion chamber for rehydration IV. If not available and supervision poor, consider NG rehydration.

Helminth infections – "worms"

Adult worms in intestine

Symptom/sign:	Suggests this worm infection:
Short stature, not growing	Trichuris or hookworm
Mild/moderate muscle wasting	Trichuris or hookworm
Anaemia, microcytic hypochromic	Hookworm or severe trichuriasis; not *Ascaris*
Hypoproteinaemia, possible oedema	Hookworm or severe trichuriasis or disseminated strongyloidiasis; not *Ascaris*
Pica, especially eating soil (geophagia)	Any or all helminths
Colicky abdominal pain	Ascaris: common but a weak correlation
Intestinal obstruction	Ascaris: quite common surgical emergency
Jaundice and/or pancreatitis	Ascaris: uncommon
Laryngeal obstruction	Ascaris: rare
Vomiting up worms	Ascaris: common
Chronic diarrhoea	Trichuris or severe hookworm or strongyloidiasis
Defaecating during sleeping hours	Trichuris
Blood and mucus in stool	Trichuris
Rectal prolapse	Trichuris
Finger clubbing	Intense trichuriasis or hookworm; not *Ascaris*
Perianal itching	Enterobius
Vulvovaginitis	Enterobius

Illness due to "larvae" rather than adult worms

Symptom/sign:	Suggests this worm infection:
Larvae in viscera	
Cough and wheeze	*Toxocara canis/cati* (dog/cat roundworm) and also *Ascaris* and hookworm
Hepatomegaly	*Toxocara*
Lymphadenopathy	*Toxocara*
Leucocytosis with extreme eosinophilia	*Toxocara*
Epilepsy/encephalopathy	*Toxocara* (rare)
Uveitis or proliferative retinitis	*Toxocara* (younger children escape in endemic areas: naive strangers are more susceptible)
Larvae in/under skin	
Itchy area with red wiggly line, moving from day to day, often with pyoderma	*Ancylostoma braziliensis* (dog hookworm)

Investigation for migrating larvae

Eosinophilia is characteristic but is a useless diagnostic marker for intestinal infection.

The chest *x* ray may show a flaring shadow spreading out from the hila.

Treatment

Mebendazole and **albendazole** are drugs of choice for ascariasis, hookworm infection, trichuriasis, and enterobiasis in children > 2 years. For children < 2 years of age piperazine 45–75 mg/kg once daily for 3 days.

Mebendazole: 100 mg and 500 mg tablets, 20 mg/5 ml liquid. Standard treatment for *Trichuris* infection or symptomatic hookworm infection is 100 mg twice daily for 3 days.

Albendazole: Superior efficacy to mebendazole in systemically invasive conditions: more effective against migrating larvae 200 mg tablets or 200 mg/5 ml liquid. Standard treatment for *Trichuris* infection is 400 mg daily for 3 days.

Environmental emergencies

Envenoming

Consider with unexplained illness, particularly if severe pain, swelling, or blistering of limb, or if bleeding or signs of neurotoxicity.

Snakebite

Local effects

Pain, swelling or blistering of the bitten limb. Necrosis at site of the wound.

Systemic effects

- Non-specific symptoms:
    vomiting, headache, collapse
    painful regional lymph node enlargement indicating absorption of venom.
- Specific signs:
    non-clotting of blood: bleeding from gums, old wounds, sores
    neurotoxicity: ptosis, bulbar palsy, and respiratory paralysis
    rhabdomyolysis: muscle pains and black urine
    shock: hypotension, usually due to hypovolaemia.

First aid

- Reassure. Many symptoms due to anxiety.
- Immobilise and splint the limb. Moving the limb may increase systemic absorption of venom.
- Wipe site with clean cloth.
- Avoid cutting/suction/tourniquets.
- Apply a pressure bandage especially if bite from snakes that cause neurotoxicity. Apply a crepe bandage over the bite site and wind firmly up the limb.

- Transport to hospital as soon as possible.
- If snake killed, take it to hospital.

Diagnosis and initial assessment (think of envenoming in unusual cases)

- Examine bitten limb for local signs.
- Watch for shock.
- Look for non-clotting blood. 20 minute whole blood clotting test (WBCT20) on admission and repeat 6 hours later.

Place a few millilitres of freshly sampled blood in a new clean dry glass tube or bottle. Leave undisturbed for 20 minutes at ambient temperature. Tip vessel once. If blood is still liquid (unclotted) and runs out, patient has hypofibrinogenaemia ("incoagulable blood") as a result or venom-induced consumption coagulopathy.

- Look for signs of bleeding (gums/old wounds/sores). Bleeding internally (most often intracranial) may cause clinical signs.
- Look for early signs of neurotoxicity; ptosis (children may interpret this as feeling sleepy), limb weakness, or difficulties in talking, swallowing, or breathing.
- Check for muscle tenderness and myoglobinuria in seasnake bites.
- Take blood for:
    Hb, WCC and platelet count
    prothrombin time, activated partial thromboplastin time (APTT), and fibrinogen levels
    serum urea and creatinine
    creatine phosphokinase (CPK) (reflecting skeletal muscle damage)
- ECG
- Observe for at least 24 hours, even if there are no signs of envenoming initially. Review regularly; envenoming may develop quite rapidly.

- Avoid IM injections and invasive procedures.
- Give tetanus prophylaxis. Routine antibiotic prophylaxis not required unless necrosis.

Antivenom

For systemic envenoming or in severe local envenoming if swelling extends more than half the bitten limb or local necrosis. Monospecific (monovalent) antivenom may be used for a single species of snake, polyspecific (polyvalent) for a number of different species. **Children require same dose as adults** (depends on amount of venom injected, **not** bodyweight).

- Dilute antivenom in 2–3 volumes of 0·9% saline and infuse over 1 hour. Infusion rate should be slow initially and gradually increased.
- Have epinephrine ready in a syringe (10 micrograms/kg).
- Observe closely during antivenom administration for adverse reaction. Common early signs urticaria and itching, restlessness, fever, cough, or feeling of constriction in the throat.
- Patients with these signs should be treated with epinephrine 10 micrograms/kg IM and if a nebuliser is available, 5 ml 1 in 1000 adrenaline. An antihistamine, for example chlorpheniramine (250 micrograms/kg IM or IV) also given.
- Unless life-threatening anaphylaxis has occurred, antivenom cautiously restarted.
- Monitor response to antivenom. In presence of coagulopathy, restoration of clotting depends upon hepatic re-synthesis of clotting factors. Repeat WBCT20 and other clotting studies if available, 6 hours after antivenom; if blood is still non-clotting, further antivenom is indicated. After restoration of normal clotting, measure clotting at 6 hourly intervals as a coagulopathy may recur due to late absorption of venom from bite.

- Response of neurotoxicity to antivenom is less predictable. In species with predominantly postsynaptically acting toxins, antivenom may reverse neurotoxicity; failure to do so is an indication for further doses. However, response to antivenom is poor in species with presynaptically acting toxins.

Other therapy

- Excise sloughs from necrotic wounds. Skin grafting may be necessary. Severe swelling may lead to suspicion of a compartment syndrome. Fasciotomy if definite evidence of raised intracompartmental pressure (> 45 mmHg) if measurable, and any coagulopathy corrected. Note: clinical assessment often misleading following snakebite, therefore objective criteria necessary.
- Blood products are not necessary to treat a coagulopathy if adequate antivenom has been given.
- Endotracheal intubation/tracheostomy if bulbar palsy develops; difficulty in swallowing leads to pooling of secretions.
- Paralysis of intercostal muscles and diaphragm requires artificial ventilation. If ventilator not available this can be performed by manual bagging (mask or ET tube) and may need to be maintained for days, using relays of relatives if necessary.
- Anticholinesterases may reverse neurotoxicity following envenoming by some species.
- Maintain careful fluid balance to treat shock and prevent renal failure.
- Some cobras spit venom into the eyes of their victims. Rapid irrigation with water will prevent severe inflammation. 0·5% epinephrine drops may help to reduce pain and inflammation.

Scorpion stings

Severe pain around bite for many hours or days. Systemic envenoming is more common in children and may occur within minutes of a bite. Major clinical features are caused by activation of the autonomic nervous system.

Clinical features

Tachypnoea	Muscle twitches and spasms
Excessive salivation	Hypertension
Nausea and vomiting	Pulmonary oedema
Lacrimation	Cardiac arrhythmias
Sweating	Hypotension
Abdominal pain	Respiratory failure

Severe hypertension, myocardial failure, and pulmonary oedema are particularly prominent in severe envenoming.

Management

- Hospital immediately; delay is a frequent cause of death.
- Control pain with infiltration of 1% lidocaine (lignocaine) around wound or IV morphine.
- Scorpion antivenom is available. Give IV/IM in systemic envenoming.
- Prazosin is effective for treating hypertension and cardiac failure (5–15 micrograms/kg 2–4 times a day increasing to control blood pressure to a maximum of 500 micrograms/kg/day). Lie down for first 4–6 hours of treatment in case of sudden fall in BP.
- Severe pulmonary oedema requires aggressive treatment with diuretics and vasodilators.

Spider bites

Widow spiders (Latrodectus spp.)
Severe pain at bite. Rarely systemic envenoming with abdominal and generalised pain and other features due to transmitter release from autonomic nerves. Hypertension is characteristic (prazosin – see above). Antivenom is available. Opiates and diazepam for pain.

Recluse spiders (Loxosceles spp.)
Bites in which pain develops over a number of hours. A white ischaemic area gradually breaks down to form a black eschar

over 7 days or so. Healing may be prolonged and occasionally severe scarring occurs.

Banana spiders (Phoneutria spp.)

Severe burning pain at bite may cause systemic envenoming with tachycardia, hypertension, sweating, and priapism. Polyspecific antivenom available.

Marine envenoming: venomous fish

Systemic envenoming is rare. Excruciating pain at site of sting is the major effect. Regional nerve blocks and local infiltration of 1% lidocaine may be effective. Most marine venoms are heat labile, immersing in hot water is effective in relieving pain. Care to avoid scalding; the envenomed limb may have abnormal sensation. Clinicians check water temperature and patient immerse the non-bitten limb as well.

Jellyfish

Rubbing sting will cause further discharge and worsen envenoming. In box jellyfish stings, pouring vinegar over the sting will prevent discharge of nematocysts. For most other jellyfish, seawater should be poured over stings and adherent tentacles gently removed. Ice is useful for pain relief. Box jellyfish stings occasionally rapidly life threatening. Antivenom is available IM.

Near drowning

- Toddlers can drown in small volumes of water, for example in a bucket or shallow pool.
- Not all drowning is accidental (abuse/neglect).
- Other injuries may be present.
- Other illnesses may have resulted in the drowning, for example epilepsy.
- Water can be fresh (hypotonic) or salt (hypertonic).
- Water can conceal hidden dangers: trauma, entrapment, tide and flow, contamination.

- Water can act as a solid at high impact velocity.
- Water may be only one of several problems afflicting the victim:

  Alcohol, drugs, child abuse, epilepsy, trauma, etc.

Problems which may be present

- Hypothermia
- Hypoxia/pulmonary oedema/adult respiratory distress syndrome (ARDS)
- Hypotension/ventricular dysrhythmias/cardiac arrest
- Cerebral depression/coma/hypoxic ischaemic brain injury
- Other injuries, especially spinal and head injuries
- Electrolyte disturbances
- Ingestions such as alcohol, anticonvulsant drugs
- Pre-existing epilepsy.

Assessment and resuscitation

Airway and cervical spine control, gastric decompression.
Breathing – intubation (with PEEP), high concentration O_2.
Circulation and control of external haemorrhage:
    feel for brachial/carotid pulse
    capillary refill time (difficult if hypothermia)
Disability and mini neurological examination (AVPU)
Exposure and temperature control – core temperature measurement (best 10 cm into rectum).

REWARMING – Beware rewarming shock; do not allow temp to rise > 37°C. Prevent further heat loss: remove cold wet clothes.

External rewarming if > 32°C with radiant heater, dry warm blankets.

Core rewarming if < 32°C:
Warmed IV fluid to 39°C
Gastric lavage with 0·9% saline at 42°C
Heated humidified oxygen (42°C).

Resuscitation should not be discontinued until the core temperature is > 32°C or cannot be raised.

Hyper- and hypothermia

Heat stroke

Clinical signs

- Confusion
- Tachycardia
- Fever (> 40°C)
- Hot dry skin
- Tachypnoea
- Hypotonia.

Treatment

Urgent cooling

- Aim to cool within 30 minutes (especially head). Remove clothes, spray with cool water, fan if available, ice packs to neck, axillae, and groins.
- Provide system support as necessary.
- Give fluids IV, especially if respiratory failure.
- Give oxygen.

Hypothermia in infants

Cold environment, malnutrition, or serious infection (low reading thermometer core (rectal) < 32°C = severe; 32–35·9°C = moderate). Alternatively if axillary temperature < 35°C or does not register assume hypothermia.

- WARM: kangaroo care with mother given warm drink or thermostatically controlled heated mattress (37–38°C) or air-heated incubator 35–36°C.
- If mother not available hot water bottle in cot **removed before infant**.
- Cover the head/dress in warm DRY clothes. Keep nappy dry.

- When examining do not allow temperature to fall (ideally room temperature should be > 25°C and no draughts).
- Feed 2 hourly and feed during the night (4 hourly).
- Avoid washing.
- Sleep with mother.

Trauma and surgical

Acute abdomen

Appendicitis
Clinical presentation

- Very variable.
- Pain always and first symptom. Early visceral pain non-specific in epigastric or umbilical region and **only later** localises over appendix. Pain with pelvic appendix delayed. Pain of retrocaecal appendix in flank or back.
- Anorexia, nausea, and vomiting within a few hours.
- Diarrhoea more frequently in children may indicate a pelvic abscess.
- **Child lies in bed with minimal movement**.
- Fever and tachycardia.
- **There may be localised tenderness at McBurney's point**.
- Auscultate chest (CXR) to exclude pneumonia.
- **Single most important issue is serial examination by same person**.
- Increase in WBC but is unreliable.
- Ultrasonography effective.

Intussusception
Clinical presentation

- Infant aged 4–12 months suddenly disturbed by violent abdominal pain which is intermittent, builds up with spasms, draws up knees, screams, becomes pale, sweats, and vomits. Seems to recover immediately and may resume normal eating habits, until stricken by another bout.
- Classically fresh bloodstained stool.
- **Pain + vomiting + blood only in a third of patients.** 1 in 10 have diarrhoea.
- Pallor, persistent apathy, and dehydration are common.

- Emptiness in right lower quadrant and **sausage-shaped mass in the right hypochondrium** extending along line of transverse colon. **Absence does not rule out intussusception**.
- Fever and leucocytosis, tachycardia and hypovolaemia.
- Abdominal x ray/mass across central abdomen with dilated loops of bowel.
- **Ultrasonography reliable**.

Intestinal obstruction

- **Extrinsic:** incarcerated hernia and vascular bands, intussusception, anomalies of rotation (volvulus and Ladds bands, paraduodenal and paracaecal hernias), postoperative adhesions.
- **Intrinsic:** inspissation of bowel contents (meconium ileus, distal intestinal obstruction syndrome in cystic fibrosis (CF), roundworm obstruction. Peristaltic dysfunction – Hirschsprung's disease. Inflammatory lesions – tuberculosis, Crohn's disease.

Clinical presentation

- Cramping abdominal pain with anorexia, nausea, and vomiting which progresses to bile stained
- Abdominal distension (greater more distal the obstruction)
- Tachycardia and dehydration
- Tenderness and hyperactive bowel sounds.

Chest and abdominal films are taken to confirm the diagnosis of obstruction and rule out the presence of free air.

Treatment

- Relieve obstruction before ischaemic bowel injury occurs.
- IV access and baseline bloods collected for baseline investigations including a full blood count, urea, creatinine and electrolytes and cross-match.
- 0·9% saline with 10% glucose 4 ml/kg/h for the first 10 kg, 2 ml/kg/h for the next 10 kg and 1 ml/kg/h for subsequent kg.

- Potassium added, once good urine output (> 1 ml/kg/h in child and > 2ml/kg/h in infant).
- Some may need one or more IV boluses (10–20 ml/kg) of 0·9% saline/4·5% albumin for resuscitation.
- NG tube for decompression.

Broad spectrum IV antibiotics such as:
- Cefuroxime 50 mg/kg 8 hourly or 12 hourly in the neonate and metronidazole 7·5 mg/kg 8 hourly given IV over 20 minutes **or**
- Benzylpenicillin 50 mg/kg 6 hourly plus gentamicin: 1 month to 12 years (6 mg/kg once daily), 12–18 years (5 mg/kg once daily) plus metronidazole.

Once patient adequately resuscitated and fluid and electrolyte imbalance safe, laparotomy is performed and the cause treated.

At all times adequate analgesia.

Life-threatening trauma

	Primary survey
A	Airway with cervical spine control
B	Breathing and ventilation
C	Circulation and haemorrhage control
D	Disability assessment
E	Exposure

Airway with cervical spine control
- Clear, unobstructed airway.
- High concentration O_2 through reservoir mask or, if breathing needs support, through self-inflating bag + O_2 reservoir.
- Where cervical spine at risk, head and neck in neutral alignment. Immediately by manual in-line immobilisation.

A correctly fitting hard collar, side-supports, and head blocks then maintain immobilisation until spine cleared. Manual in-line method resumed if airway manoeuvres such as intubation. Normal x rays do **not** exclude spinal cord injury.

Signs of airway obstruction:

- Rapid rate
- Noisy breathing (total obstruction may be silent)
- Recession/paradoxical breathing
- Cyanosis
- Agitation or drowsiness
- Decreased or absent breath sounds on auscultation.

The airway should be cleared of debris and careful jaw thrust applied. If no improvement oropharyngeal airway inserted.

If still obstructed: orotracheal intubation under direct vision with manual in-line stabilisation of the cervical spine

- Pre-oxygenation with 100% oxygen with manual lung inflation if required
- Administration of a carefully judged, reduced dose of an anaesthetic induction agent
- Application of cricoid pressure
- Suxamethonium 1–2 mg/kg
- Intubation with a correctly sized tracheal tube
- Replacement of the collar and blocks after confirming tube placement and relaxing cricoid pressure.

Confirmation of correct placement of the tube

Most important see tube pass through vocal cords. The correct size is tube placed easily through cords with small leak. Place tube 2–3 cm below cords and note length at teeth before check by auscultation. If orotracheal intubation not possible, needle cricothyroidotomy or in > 11 years surgical cricothyroidotomy.

Breathing – assessment of adequacy of respiration

- Rate
- Chest expansion
- Recession
- Use of accessory muscles
- Nasal flaring
- Inspiratory or expiratory noises
- Breath sounds
- Heart rate
- Colour
- Mental state
- Pulse oximetry.

Examine trachea, neck veins, and chest for pleural collections of air or blood. Tension pneumothorax treated immediately with needle thoracocentesis in 2nd intercostal space on affected side in midclavicular line, followed by tube thoracostomy.

Circulatory assessment

- Capillary refill
- Skin colour
- Temperature
- Systolic blood pressure
- Mental state
- Respiratory rate.

The blood pressure is initially well maintained despite continuing bleeding, due to child's exceptional ability to vasoconstrict. As indicator of haemorrhage, normal BP can be falsely reassuring; a tachycardia more revealing. For obvious external haemorrhage controlled manual pressure.

- Cannulate peripheral vein
- Intraosseous infusion
- Femoral vein catheterisation   } avoid if pelvic/
- Venous cutdown (saphenous vein)   } abdominal injury
- Jugular or subclavian vein catheterisation.

Blood typing, cross-matching, haemoglobin and full blood count, glucose and electrolytes.

Bolus of 20 ml/kg of warmed 0·9% saline or Hartmann's. Repeat twice, after this consider surgical intervention and transfusion. **The most important aspect of fluid resuscitation is the child's response to the fluid challenge**. Improvement is indicated by:

- Decrease in heart rate
- Increase in skin temperature
- Quicker capillary refill
- Improving mental state
- Increase in systolic blood pressure
- Satisfactory urine output.

If fail to improve carry out urgent search for chest, abdominal, or pelvic haemorrhage.

Give initial fluid bolus by attaching warmed fluid bag to IV cannula via three-way tap and 20 mL syringe and administer sequentially the same number of syringe-fulls (as the number of kg body wt of child)

Disability

AVPU plus pupil size and reactivity and Glasgow Coma Scale.

Exposure

Undress (use scissors to cut clothes) for anatomical search for injuries. **Avoid prolonged exposure**.

At end of primary survey, the severely injured child should have:

Clear airway, breathing 100% oxygen

Cervical spine immobilisation in blunt trauma cases

Adequate respiration, achieved by manual or mechanical ventilation and chest decompression when indicated

Venous access and an initial fluid challenge if indicated on circulatory assessment

Blood sent for typing and cross-matching

The potential need for immediate life-saving surgery considered and preparations
underway

The following life-threatening conditions excluded or identified and treated:

	Treatment
Airway obstruction	Intubation or surgical airway
Tension pneumothorax	Needle thoracocentesis, chest drain
Open pneumothorax	Chest drain, 3 sided dressing
Massive haemothorax	Chest drain/blood transfusion
Flail chest	Intubation if large
Cardiac tamponade	Pericardiocentesis

Adjuncts:

ECG/oxygen saturation/blood pressure monitoring

Gastric and urinary catheters

X rays of the chest and pelvis – and cervical spine

Ultrasound scan of the abdomen

Adequate pain control

Careful titration of IV opioids (GREAT CARE IF HEAD INJURED)

Secondary survey

Examination head-to-toe, including *the back, avoiding spinal movement* (by log rolling). Document all injuries.

- Thorough re-examination of the chest front and back, using the classical *inspection–palpation–percussion–auscultation* approach, is combined with a chest *x* ray.
- Symmetry of chest movement and breath sounds, presence of surgical emphysema, and pain or instability on compressing the chest.
- Tracheal deviation and altered heart sounds are noted.

- On log-rolling reconsider **flail chest** as a posterior floating segment is often poorly tolerated.

Abdomen is *silent* area. Must be actively *cleared* of injury. Cardiovascular decompensation may occur late and precipitously.

- Thorough history taking and a careful examination of the abdomen may give clues to the origin of bleeding or perforation.
- **Gastric distension** may cause respiratory embarrassment and a **gastric tube** should be placed.
- In a severely injured child, a **urinary catheter** should be inserted, unless there is pelvic injury, examining first urine for red blood cells.
- Abdominal ultrasound and CT scanning.

Management of spinal cord injuries (SCI)

- Contain "biomechanical instability" by preventing movement at fracture.
- Dexamethasone in all acute SCI (500 micrograms/kg stat then 50 micrograms/kg every 6 hours for 48 hours).
- "Rehabilitation" as soon as possible.

Emergency treatment of traumatic amputation

- Partial or complete amputation.
- Greater blood loss with partial amputation – partially transected blood vessels do not go into spasm (as do transected vessels).
- A thorough history concerning bleeding from the limb is crucial.
- Control of exsanguinating haemorrhage is essential
    if local pressure + elevation unsuccessful, apply a tourniquet

use a broad tourniquet rather than a narrow one

place as close to the amputation as possible

pneumatic tourniquets or a BP cuff are best – inflate to above arterial pressure.

- Always record time of tourniquet inflation/application. Check every 10–15 mins: if bleeding controllable with pressure, release tourniquet. Never use tourniquet for > 2 hours.
- Good rapid fluid resuscitation is necessary.
- Urgent orthopaedic or plastic surgical help is necessary.
- Adequate analgesia, usually an opiate.
- Reimplantation of amputated limb may be possible.
- Amputated limb viable for 8 hours at room temperature.
- Amputated limb viable for 18 hours if kept sterile and in ice (avoid direct contact between ice and skin).
- **Amputated limb and child must be transported in the same vehicle.**

Gunshot wounds

Initial measures

Similar to those for any severe injury:

- General assessment and resuscitation, addressing potentially life-threatening conditions according to ABC priorities (airway, breathing, stopping haemorrhage).
- Application of dressings to open wounds.
- Emergency splintage of fractures.
- Obtaining intravenous access.
- The degree to which fluid resuscitation should be carried out is controversial. Advanced trauma life support (ATLS) teaching recommends an initial bolus of 20 ml/kg, after which the child should be carefully monitored with respect to the adequacy of organ perfusion and the response to this initial fluid challenge.
- Analgesia as required.
- Antibiotics – the ICRC recommend benzylpenicillin IV at a dose appropriate to the size of the child. (50 mg/kg IV 6 hourly).

- Tetanus toxoid and antitetanus serum.
- Appropriate radiographs of the injured areas.

Wound excision

Removal of any dead and contaminated tissue which if left would become a medium for infection.

Management of burns

- Protect airway.
- Consider other injuries?
- Expose and assess burn area. (See figure below.)
- If > 10%, establish IV line and give IV analgesia (morphine 100 micrograms/kg loading dose).
- Commence 0·9% saline or Hartmann's at 2–4 ml/kg per % burn for first 24 hours, backdated to time of burn. Half (in hourly divided doses) during the first 8 hours, and second half in next 16 hours (in hourly doses) adjusted to urine output and cardiovascular response.
- Assess area of burn and draw on chart.
- It is common to overestimate the size of burn.
- Erythema MUST NOT be included – fluid is not lost.
- An overestimation will mean that far too much fluid given.

First aid – cold water

Seconds count. Except with electricity, cold water/milk applied immediately and for 10 minutes before clothes removed. Then cover with clean dressings or cling film. Following above, avoid hypothermia, especially in babies.

ABC

- In severe burns all vascular bed leaky.
- If < 10% replace orally. If vomiting IV fluids. If safe IV access is not available, then burns of up to 25% can be managed with increased oral fluids. Small regular doses.
- For oral fluids, ORS ideal

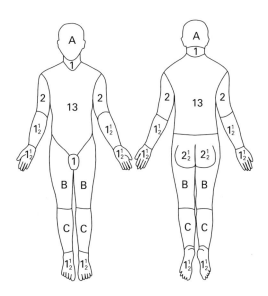

% surface area				
Age	0	1yr	5yr	10yr	15yr
A	9·5	8·5	6·5	5·5	4·5
B	2·75	3·25	4·0	4·5	4·5
C	2·5	2·5	2·75	3·0	3·25

- Hot water burns (scalds) may be superficial or deep dermal. Flame or hot fat almost always deep.
- The appearance can be altered by first aid treatments.
- First – assess capillary return.
- Second – test sensation. Is it increased (in a superficial partial thickness burn), reduced (in a deep dermal burn),

or absent (in a full thickness burn). Sterile hypodermic
needle. Difference between sharp and blunt ends. In young
children when sleeping.

- Many superficial burns become deeper during first 48 hours.

Intravenous fluids

- Ideally by peripheral vein; in emergency, intraosseous, or
  central venous lines may be needed but increase risk of
  infection.
- DO NOT USE long lines – increased risk of septicaemia.
- 0·9% saline is the best IV fluid plus 5–10% glucose in child
  < 2 years.

Natural colloids, i.e. 4·5% albumin, plasma, and blood,
artificial colloids, i.e Haemaccel and Gelofusine plus
crystalloids can be used. Excessive IV fluid may lead to
pulmonary and/or cerebral oedema, together with excessive
extravascular deposition of fluid including "compartment
syndrome".

- Fluid loss decreases 48–72 hours after injury.
- Accurate and updated fluid input and output charts are
  kept + daily weighing.
- For > 30% burns hourly haematocrit (or haemoglobin) and
  urine outputs (ideally > 1 ml/kg/h) are helpful in the first
  24 hours and then decreasing afterwards. For burns
  between 10% and 30% hourly tests.
- > 30% burns and involving the genitalia and in young
  normally incontinent female children, a urinary catheter is
  essential. In males, a urinary bag can be used.

Enteral fluids

- For 5–10% burns, daily requirement increased by 50% to
  allow for the burn (given on an hourly basis).
- The normal oral requirement of a child can be calculated
  as 100 ml/kg for the first 10 kg, 50 ml/kg for the next 10 kg,
  and 20 ml/kg for any weight up to the total weight of
  the child per 24 hours.

- This may need to be increased by 10% or 20% in hot climates.
- For example, in a child of 1 year old where the daily requirement is 800 ml, add 400 ml (i.e. 50% extra) for the burn making 1200 ml, divide by 24 and thus give 50 ml orally per hour.
- Use ORS or diluted milk or water.
- Early feeding reduces gastric ulcer formation. A thin bore NG tube can be used to give milk or other similar high protein foodstuffs.
- IV feeding is strongly contraindicated.

Dressings

- Establish and update antitetanus status.
- Consider an escharotomy.
- Dress the burned areas, or treat any area which is going to be kept exposed (give adequate analgesia: morphine, ketamine or entonox).
- Burn wound is usually sterile.
- Hands washed and sterile gloves used by all members of the team. Ideally plastic aprons.

Dressings used:

To maintain sterility

To relieve pain

To absorb fluid produced by the burn wound

To aid healing

- The layer of the dressing closest to the wound should contain an antiseptic: chlorhexidine or iodine.
- On top of this dressing should be placed a layer of gauze and then sterile cotton wool to absorb fluid.
- The whole to be held in place by a bandage.

Procedures and equipment

AIRWAY

Intubation

- Uncuffed < 25 kg. Larynx narrowest at cricoid ring.
- Correct tube is that which passes easily through the glottis and subglottic area with a small air leak detectable at 20 cm water (= sustained gentle positive pressure).
- Size of tube is one that can just fit into the nostril.
- In preterm neonates 2·5–3·5 mm internal diameter.
- In fullterm neonates 3·0–4·0 mm internal diameter.
- In infants after neonatal period 3·5 to 4·5 mm internal diameter.
- In children over 1 year = age/4 + 4 internal diameter in mm.
- Length of tube in cm = age (in years)/2 plus 12 for oral tube, = age (in years)/2 plus 15 for nasal tube.

Aids to intubation

- Laryngoscope: blade (straight for neonates and infants, curved for older children), check bulb and handle
- Magill forceps
- Introducer (not further than end of tube itself)
- Gum elastic bougie (over which tube can pass)
- Cricoid pressure (can help visualisation of larynx)
- Suction.

Predicting difficulty

Likely to be difficult:	Difficulty in opening mouth
	Reduced neck mobility
	Laryngeal/pharyngeal lesions
Congenital:	Pierre–Robin, mucopolysaccharoidoses
Acquired:	Burns, trauma
Look from side:	small chin = difficult

- Choose appropriate tube size with one size above and below.
- Get tape ready.

- Suction.
- Induce anaesthesia and give muscle relaxant unless completely obtunded.

Do not attempt in semiconscious child

Procedure

Position

- > 3–4 years: "sniffing" position (head extended on shoulders, flexed at neck, pillow under head).
- < 3 years (especially neonates and infants): neutral position (large occiput).
- Keep in neutral position with in-line immobilisation if unstable cervical spine (trauma, Down's).

Oxygenate child

- Introduce laryngoscope into right side of mouth.
- Sweep tongue to the left.
- Advance blade until epiglottis seen.
- Curved blade: advance blade anterior to epiglottis; lift epiglottis forward by moving blade away from own body.
- Straight blade: advance blade beneath epiglottis, into oesophagus; pull back, glottis will "flop" into view.

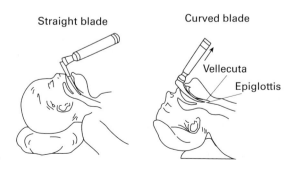

Straight blade   Curved blade

Vellecuta

Epiglottis

Recognise glottis

- Insert endotracheal tube gently through vocal cords.
- Stop at predetermined length (2–3 cm in).

Confirm correct placement

- Chest moves adequately and each side equally with ventilation.
- Listen to breath sounds in axillae and anterior chest wall.
- Confirm no breath sounds in stomach. Confirm no air bubbling back through throat.
- Oxygen saturations do not go down.
- Carbon dioxide measured from expired gases (ideal).
- CXR

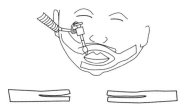

Secure tube

Proceed to nasal intubation if skilled (for long term ventilation). Two strips of sticky zinc oxide tape to reach from in front of ear across cheek and above upper lip to opposite ear.

- If available, apply benzoin tincture to cheeks, above upper lip, and under chin (to make tape stick better).
- Start with the broad end of the tape: stick this onto the cheek, then wrap one of the thinner ends carefully around the tube. It is useful still being able to see the ET tube marking at the lips.
- The other half gets taped across philtrum to the cheek.
- The second tape starts on the other cheek, and the thinner half gets stuck across the chin, the other half also wrapped around the tube.

Emergency surgical airway

< 12 years needle cricothyroidotomy; > 12 years surgical cricothyroidotomy.

In a small infant, or if foreign body below cricoid, direct tracheal puncture using the same technique.

Needle cricothyroidotomy (sterile technique)

- Attach cricothyroidotomy cannula-over-needle (or IV cannula and needle 16–18G) size to 5 ml syringe.
- Supine.
- If no risk of cervical spine injury, extend neck, with roll under shoulders.

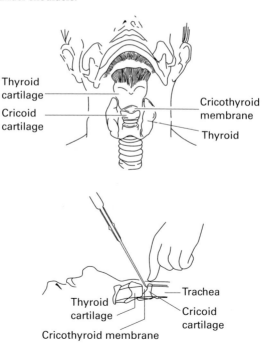

- Identify cricothyroid membrane by palpation between thyroid and cricoid cartilages.
- Stabilise the cricothyroid membrane.
- Insert cannula through cricothyroid membrane at 45 degree angle caudally, aspirating as advanced.
- When air aspirated advance cannula over needle, care with posterior tracheal wall. Withdraw the needle.
- Re-check air can be aspirated.
- Attach cannula to an oxygen flowmeter via a Y-connector. Oxygen flow rate (in litres) set to age (in years).
- Ventilate by occluding open end of Y-connector with thumb for 1 second. If chest does not rise increase oxygen flow rate by increments of 1 litre, and the effect of 1 second's occlusion of the Y-connector reassessed.
- Allow passive exhalation (via the upper airway) by taking the thumb off for 4 seconds.
- Observe chest movement and auscultate breath sounds to confirm adequate ventilation. Check the neck to exclude swelling from injection of gas into tissues.
- Proceed to tracheotomy.

Important notes

Not possible to ventilate with self-inflating bag. The maximum pressure from bag is 45 cmH$_2$O (the blow-off valve pressure), which is insufficient to drive gas through a narrow cannula. Expiration cannot occur through cannula. Expiration must occur via the upper airway, even if partial upper airway obstruction. Should upper airway obstruction be complete, reduce gas flow to 1–2 L/min to provide oxygenation but little ventilation.

Surgical cricothyroidotomy

- > 12 years.
- Supine position.
- If no risk of neck injury, extend the neck. Otherwise, maintain neutral alignment.

- Identify cricothyroid membrane.
- Prepare the skin and, if conscious, local anaesthetic.
- Stabilise the cricothyroid membrane.
- Small vertical incision in the skin, and press the lateral edges of the incision outwards, to minimise bleeding.
- Transverse incision through the cricothyroid membrane, being careful not to damage the cricoid cartilage.
- Insert tracheal spreader, or use handle of scalpel by inserting it through the incision and twisting it 90 degrees to open the airway.
- Insert endotracheal or tracheostomy tube (slightly smaller than used for oral or nasal tube).
- Ventilate patient and check effective.
- Secure tube.

BREATHING

Emergency Needle Thoracocentesis

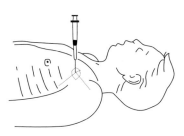

Followed by chest drain (sterile technique).
- Large over-needle IV cannula (16G or 20–22G in preterm).
- Identify 2nd intercostal space (ICS) in midclavicular line (MCL) line on side of pneumothorax (*opposite* side to direction of tracheal deviation).
- Attach the syringe to the cannula.
- Insert the cannula vertically into chest wall, just above surface of the rib below the 2nd ICS, aspirating all the time.

- If air aspirated, remove needle, leave cannula, tape in place, and proceed to chest drain insertion.

*If needle thoracocentesis is attempted, and tension pneumothorax not present, the chance of **causing** pneumothorax is 10–20%. Perform CXR.*

Insertion of chest drain (sterile technique/local anaesthesia and morphine)

Largest size drain that passes between ribs.

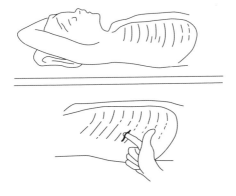

Procedure

- Prepare underwater seal and take sterile end, ready to connect to chest tube once inserted.
- Cover underwater end of tube by no more than 1–2 cmH$_2$O.
- Insertion site (usually 4th–5th ICS in anterior or midaxillary line).
- Make 1–3 cm skin incision along the line of ICS, **immediately above the rib below to avoid damage to**

the neurovascular bundle which lies under the inferior edge of each rib.

- Bluntly dissect using artery forceps just over top of the rib below, and puncture parietal pleura with the tip of the forceps.
- Put a gloved finger into the incision and clear the path into the pleura (not possible in small children).
- Holding the chest drain about 1 cm from the end pass it into the hole you have made – it should thread in easily.
- Pass about 3 cm, more if bigger child and draining haemothorax, connect to underwater seal.
- Ensure tube is in pleural space by listening for air movement, and by looking for fogging of the tube during expiration.
- Secure the tube using a suture passed through the skin at the incision site (ensure adequate local anaesthetic) and tied around the tube.
- Cover the puncture site in the chest wall with a sterile dressing and tape the chest tube to the chest wall – cotton gauze under "Opsite" may provide an optimal occlusive dressing.
- CXR.

If the chest tube is working, occasional bubbles will pass through the underwater seal. The water level in the tube may also rise and fall slightly with the respiratory cycle.

Pleural tap for effusion

CXR. If confirms – diagnostic tap.

- Child on mother's lap, facing her, held tightly in bear hug.
- 5th intercostal space on the superior aspect of the 6th rib in the mid-axillary line just below nipple level.
- 20g needle on syringe and three-way tap, below where percussion note becomes dull. Just above the rib (to avoid blood vessels) and aspirate all the time. Avoid liver.

- Send for microscopy, protein level, cell count, gram and Ziehl–Neelsen stain, and culture for bacteria including TB. Aspirate as much fluid as possible. Ensure air does not enter.

Chest drain for empyema

Insert as sterile procedure:
- Position child and locate empyema.
- Use sufficient 1% lidocaine (lignocaine).
- Make incision in skin, stretch it to accommodate tube size firmly, and part underlying muscle with artery forceps.
- Avoid neurovascular bundle on inferior part of the rib and pass drain on top of rib.
- Puncture the pleura with forceps and thread the largest chest drain that will go between ribs. Do not use trochar as this can damage lung and large vessels.
- Ensure all drain holes of catheter are inside chest.
- Fix drain with gauze dressing, tape, and a suture.
- Connect to underwater seal. Fluid will flow out and level will "swing" with respiration.

CIRCULATION

External jugular vein (sterile technique)

- Place in 15–30° head-down position.
- Turn head away from site of puncture. Restrain with blanket below neck.
- External jugular vein passes over sternomastoid junction middle and lower thirds.
- Assistant places finger at lower end of visible part of the vein just above the clavicle.

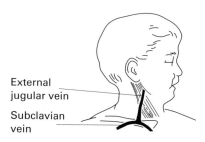

External
jugular vein

Subclavian
vein

Femoral cannulation (sterile technique)

- Supine leg slightly abducted. Towel under buttocks.
- Find femoral artery 2 cm below midpoint of inguinal ligament. Femoral vein lies immediately medial to artery. Infiltrate the skin with local anaesthetic.
- With finger on femoral artery introduce needle with syringe attached at 45 degrees to the skin along line of vein pointing towards umbilicus. Advance needle whilst aspirating.
- When blood "flashes back" into syringe remove syringe from needle, feed Seldinger guidewire through the needle holding wire at all times.

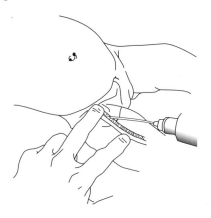

Internal jugular (sterile technique)

Head down increases vein distension and reduces risk of air embolism.

- 30 degrees head down, and turn head to left hand side for the right sided approach which avoids lymphatic duct. Place towel under shoulders to extend neck.
- Identify apex of triangle formed by two heads of the sternomastoid and clavicle and infiltrate local anaesthetic (if conscious). Alternatively identify carotid medial to sternomastoid at level of lower border of thyroid cartilage, vein is just lateral to this (usually); aim needle at 30 degrees to skin and towards the ipsilateral nipple (in infants neck is very short and vein is superficial). Estimate the length of catheter from the skin entry to the nipple.
- Direct needle at 30 degrees to the skin pointing towards the ipsilateral nipple and puncture the skin at the apex of the triangle.

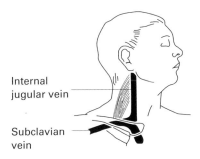

Internal jugular vein

Subclavian vein

- Advance needle, aspirating. If blood "flashes back" stop advancing, remove syringe. (If you do not cannulate vein, withdraw the needle (but not out of the skin) and advance again slightly more laterally.)
- Feed the Seldinger guidewire through the needle, always holding end of wire.

- Do not leave catheter open – risk of air embolism.
- CXR to check for a pneumothorax catheter tip at the SVC/RA junction, but not in RA.

Subclavian (sterile technique)

- Place supine, turn head to contralateral side, roll under shoulders to extend neck, identify midpoint clavicle.
- Aim for suprasternal notch, pass needle just beneath clavicle at midpoint (more medial in older child), vein lies anterior to the subclavian artery and is closest at the medial end of the clavicle.
- Subclavian artery puncture not uncommon (cannot compress to stop bleeding but rarely problem unless coagulopathy).

Cut down venous cannulation (sterile technique)

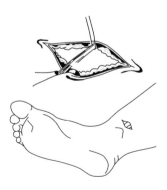

Procedure
Identify landmarks.

Brachial

Infant – one finger breadth lateral to the medial epicondyle of the humerus.

Small child – two finger breadths lateral to the medial epicondyle of the humerus.

Older child – three finger breadths lateral to the medial epicondyle of the humerus.

Saphenous

Infant – half a finger breadth superior and anterior to the medial malleolus.

Small child – one finger breadth superior and anterior to the medial malleolus.

Older child – two finger breadths superior and anterior to the medial malleolus.

- Apply tourniquet at pressure between venous and arterial.
- Local anaesthetic after marking site of vein (if conscious).
- Incise perpendicular to long axis of vein.
- Bluntly dissect subcutaneous tissues with curved artery forceps (tips pointing downwards) parallel to the vein. With tips pointing up scoop up the tissues and open the forceps – you should have picked up the vein. Clear 2 cm of vein from surrounding tissue.
- Pass proximal and distal ligature around vein. Tie the distal ligature and use for traction.
- Make small hole in vein with scalpel proximal to tied ligature and feed catheter into the vein proximally (ideally to hub). Tie proximal ligature around vein and catheter.
- Aspirate blood (if blood does not aspirate you may be against vein wall so pull back a little and repeat) and flush with normal saline. Release tourniquet.
- Close incision with interrupted sutures, place antiseptic ointment (for example, iodine) over wound, and suture the catheter to the skin (ensure local anaesthetic at suture site if conscious). Cover with dressing.

Umbilical vein catheterisation (sterile technique)

Possible < 7 days of age.

5FG (8FG in full term) umbilical catheter (sterile feeding tube may be used but first measure length. Cannulae for UVC usually marked every 5 cm).

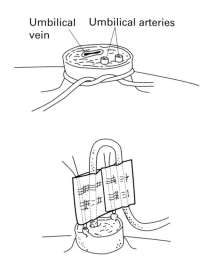

Umbilical vein   Umbilical arteries

Procedure (aseptic)

- Assemble the syringe, three-way tap, and catheter. Flush and fill catheter with sterile 0.9% saline and close tap to prevent air embolus.
- Clean the umbilical cord and surrounding skin with 0.5% chlorhexidine or 10% povidone-iodine. Tie cord ligature/tape loosely round base of cord.
- Cut back cord to about 1–2 cm from base (clean stroke of scalpel not sawing).

- Hold cord near vein with artery forceps.
- Identify the vein – usually gaping, larger, and well separated from the two small thicker-walled arteries. Grip wall of vein.
- Hold the catheter approximately 2 cm from the end with forceps and insert tip into vein. Gently advance the catheter which must pass easily. Insert for 4–6 cm for resuscitation or exchange transfusion.
- For long term use place above diaphragm at SVC/RA junction (($2 \times$ weight in kg) + 5 + length of stump in centimetres (length usually equal to distance of umbilicus to internipple line)). Check draw back blood easily – if not withdraw slightly until blood flows.
- Ideally CXR to check position; must not be in liver.
- Occasionally umbilical vein is kinked and advance of catheter is blocked at 1–2 cm beyond the abdominal wall. Gentle traction on the cord usually relieves this.
- If obstruction occurs at > 2 cm, catheter probably wedged in portal system or coiled up in the portal sinus. Withdraw part way and re-insert.
- Secure by placing two silk stitches into cord, tie, then cut 5 cm long. Line up with catheter and tape (see figure above).
- After removal apply pressure to umbilical stump for 5–10 minutes.

Exchange transfusion (sterile technique essential)

Use O–ve or blood cross-matched against *maternal* antibodies use fresh whole blood < 48 hours. Ideally warm blood (especially for low birthweight or preterm infants).

- Check blood glucose before and during exchange. Take blood for Coombs' and G6PD level.
- Although K^+ level in transfused blood = 8–10 mmol/L, does not usually cause significant hyperkalemia.
- Plan *2-hours* + observer to monitor baby and record each aliquot withdrawn and replaced.

- Connect three-way tap to the umbilical vein catheter – syringe on one, one to donor blood infusion set and another to waste bottle.
- Exchange volumes:
    < 1500 g 5 ml
    1500–2500 g 5–10 ml
    > 2500 g 10–15 ml
    aim for double volume exchange: 80 ml/kg × 2
    aim for end Hb of 15 g/dl.
- For small aliquots remember allowance for "dead space" in tubing between the syringe and the baby.
- Draw out each aliquot over 2–3 minutes and replace over 3–4 minutes.
- First aliquot for bilirubin, electrolyte, and calcium.
- Halfway through the procedure check the blood glucose, calcium, and potassium concentrations.
- Measure them again, + bilirubin, at end.

Intraosseous needle insertion (sterile technique essential)

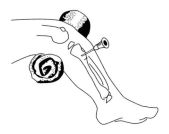

- Flat anteromedial surface of tibia, 2–3 cm below tibial tuberosity or anterolateral surface of femur, 3 cm above the lateral condyle. (Avoid bones with fractures proximal to the insertion site.)
- Position knee flexed at 30 degrees over a towel. Grasp the limb firmly.

- Insert needle 90 degrees to skin with rotating action. Feel sudden "give" as enter medulla. The needle should stand up by itself.
- Withdraw trochar and aspirate with 5 ml syringe to confirm position. Send aspirate for cross-matching of blood if needed. Flush with 0·9% saline to expel clots and observe for subcutaneous swelling. Infuse fluid boluses with 20 ml syringe.
- Secure IV access. Remove as soon as possible.

Needle pericardiocentesis (sterile technique and local anaesthetic if needed)

- Supine and attach ECG.
- Attach 16–20G cannula to the syringe. Insert cannula just below and to left of xiphoid process. Angle needle 45 degrees to skin and point to tip of left scapula.
- Advance needle, aspirating and watching cardiac monitor. As enter distended pericardial sac, fluid flows back into syringe. If myocardium is touched ECG pattern will change (arrhythmia, ectopics, "injury" pattern). If aspirate bright red blood entered ventricle; therefore withdraw slightly.

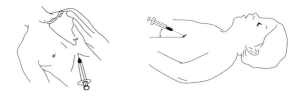

- If successful, cardiac function should improve. Withdraw needle, attach three-way tap and secure cannula for further aspiration.

Defibrillation

Basic life support interrupted for shortest possible time (5–9 below).

1. Apply gel pads or electrode gel
2. Select correct paddles (paediatric paddles for < 10 kg)
3. Select energy
4. Place the electrodes and apply firm pressure
5. Press charge button. Wait until charged
6. Shout "Stand back!"
7. Check other rescuers are clear
8. Deliver shock.

One paddle over apex in midaxillary line, other to right of sternum, immediately below clavicle. **Good paddle contact:** gel pads or electrode gel (if gel, *care* not to join two *areas of application*). Firm pressure to paddles.

Correct energy selection: 2 J/kg for first 2 shocks and then 4 J/kg.

Appendix

Adapted from WHO/NCHS normalised reference weight-for-length (50–84 cm) and weight-for-height (86–110 cm), by sex

Boys' weight (kg)					Length (cm)	Girls' weight (kg)				
-4 SD 60%	-3 SD 70%	-2 SD 80%	-1 SD 90%	Median		Median	-1 SD 90%	-2 SD 80%	-3 SD 70%	-4 SD 60%
1.8	2.2	2.5	2.9	3.3	50.0	3.4	3.0	2.6	2.3	1.9
1.9	2.3	2.8	3.2	3.7	52.0	3.7	3.3	2.8	2.4	2.0
2.0	2.6	3.1	3.6	4.1	54.0	4.1	3.6	3.1	2.7	2.2
2.3	2.9	3.5	4.0	4.6	56.0	4.5	4.0	3.5	3.0	2.4
2.7	3.3	3.9	4.5	5.1	58.0	5.0	4.4	3.9	3.3	2.7
3.1	3.7	4.4	5.0	5.7	60.0	5.5	4.9	4.3	3.7	3.1
3.5	4.2	4.9	5.6	6.2	62.0	6.1	5.4	4.8	4.1	3.5
4.0	4.7	5.4	6.1	6.8	64.0	6.7	6.0	5.3	4.6	3.9
4.5	5.3	6.0	6.7	7.4	66.0	7.3	6.5	5.8	5.1	4.3
5.1	5.8	6.5	7.3	8.0	68.0	7.8	7.1	6.3	5.5	4.8
5.5	6.3	7.0	7.8	8.5	70.0	8.4	7.6	6.8	6.0	5.2
6.0	6.8	7.5	8.3	9.1	72.0	8.9	8.1	7.2	6.4	5.6
6.4	7.2	8.0	8.8	9.6	74.0	9.4	8.5	7.7	6.8	6.0
6.8	7.6	8.4	9.2	10.0	76.0	9.8	8.9	8.1	7.2	6.4
7.1	8.0	8.8	9.7	10.2	78.0	10.2	9.3	8.5	7.6	6.7
7.5	8.3	9.2	10.1	10.9	80.0	10.6	9.7	8.8	8.0	7.1
7.8	8.7	9.6	10.4	11.3	82.0	11.0	10.1	9.2	8.3	7.4
8.1	9.0	9.9	10.8	11.7	84.0	11.4	10.5	9.6	8.7	7.7

Continued

Continued

Boys' weight (kg)					Length (cm)	Median	Girls' weight (kg)			
−4 SD 60%	−3 SD 70%	−2 SD 80%	−1 SD 90%	Median			−1 SD 90%	−2 SD 80%	−3 SD 70%	−4 SD 60%
8·3	9·4	10·5	11·7	12·8	88·0	12·5	11·4	10·3	9·2	8·1
8·6	9·8	10·9	12·1	13·3	90·0	12·9	11·8	10·7	9·5	8·4
8·9	10·1	11·3	12·5	13·7	92·0	13·4	12·2	11·0	9·9	8·7
9·2	10·5	11·7	13·0	14·2	94·0	13·9	12·6	11·4	10·2	9·0
9·6	10·9	12·1	13·4	14·7	96·0	14·3	13·1	11·8	10·6	9·3
9·9	11·2	12·6	13·9	15·2	98·0	14·9	13·5	12·2	10·9	9·6
10·3	11·6	13·0	14·4	15·7	100·0	15·4	14·0	12·7	11·3	9·9
10·6	12·0	13·4	14·9	16·3	102·0	15·9	14·5	13·1	11·7	10·3
11·0	12·4	13·9	15·4	16·9	104·0	16·5	15·0	13·5	12·1	10·6
11·4	12·9	14·4	15·9	17·4	106·0	17·0	15·5	14·0	12·5	11·0
11·8	13·4	14·9	16·5	18·0	108·0	17·6	16·1	14·5	13·0	11·4
12·2	13·8	15·4	17·1	18·7	110·0	18·2	16·6	15·0	13·4	11·9

Notes:

1. SD = standard deviation score or Z-score; although the interpretation of a fixed percent-of-median value varies across age and height, and generally, the two scales cannot be compared, the approximate percent-of-median values for −1 and −2 SD are 90% and 80% of median, respectively (*Bulletin of the World Health Organisation*, 1994, **72**:273–283).

2. Length is measured below 85 cm; height is measured 85 cm and above. Recumbent length is on average 0·5 cm greater than standing height, although the difference is of no importance to the individual child. A correction may be made by deducting 0·5 cm from all lengths above 84·9 cm if the standing height cannot be measured.

Estimating body surface area

weight kg	SA m²	weight kg	SA m²	weight kg	SA m²
0·7	0·07	12·0	0·56	38·0	1·23
1·0	0·10	13·0	0·59	40·0	1·27
1·6	0·14	14·0	0·62	42·0	1·32
2·0	0·16	15·0	0·65	44·0	1·36
2·6	0·19	16·0	0·68	46·0	1·40
3·0	0·21	17·0	0·71	48·0	1·44
3·6	0·24	18·0	0·74	50·0	1·48
4·0	0·26	19·0	0·77	52·0	1·52
4·5	0·28	20·0	0·79	54·0	1·56
5·0	0·30	22·0	0·85	56·0	1·60
5·5	0·33	24·0	0·90	58·0	1·63
6·0	0·35	26·0	0·95	60·0	1·67
7·0	0·38	28·0	1·00	65·0	1·76
8·0	0·42	30·0	1·05	70·0	1·85
9·0	0·46	32·0	1·09	75·0	1·94
10·0	0·49	34·0	1·14	80·0	2·03
11·0	0·53	36·0	1·19	90·0	2·19

Mid Upper Arm Circumference

- Non-stretchable tape midway between elbow and shoulder
- The tape tightened but not compress underlying tissues
- Child 1–5 yrs little increase. Normal 14–16 cm.

Moderate Malnutrition 12·5 to 14 cm.
Severe Malnutrition < 12·5 cm.

Management of Pain

Strong Opioid for
moderate to
severe pain
+/– Non-opioid
+/– Adjuvants

STEP 3

Weak Opioid for mild
to moderate pain
+/– Non-opioid
+/– Adjuvants

STEP 2

Non-opioid

+/– Adjuvants

STEP 1

WHO three-step analgesic ladder

Side effects of morphine

- **Respiratory depression.**

  *ALERT MEDICAL STAFF AND ENSURE NALOXONE IS
  AVAILABLE*

  Monitor SaO_2 with pulse oximeter as appropriate (SaO_2
  SHOULD NOT BE < 94% IN AIR)

- **Constipation therefore use prophylactic DOCUSATE
  SODIUM or other laxative**

CAUTION with head injuries/liver/renal impairment.

Naloxone to reverse respiratory depression =
10 micrograms/kg immediately available. (Neonatal ampoule
40 micrograms/2 ml OR adult ampoule 400 micrograms/1 ml.)
Give IV (SC or IM if not possible). Repeat after 2–3 minutes if
no response when second dose may need to be much higher
(up to 100 micrograms/kg). An IV infusion may be needed if
protracted depression of respiration occurs.

Oral analgesia for mild or moderate pain

Drug	Preparation	Comments
Paracetamol	Oral suspension 120 mg/5 ml 250 mg/5 ml	The maximum daily dose should not be given for > 3 days
ORAL loading dose 25 mg/kg Maintenance dose 20 mg/kg 6 hourly Maximum dose 80 mg/kg/24 h (60 mg/kg < 3 months)	Tablets/soluble 500 mg	Caution with liver impairment
RECTAL loading dose 40 mg/kg (20 mg/kg if < 3 months) Maintenance dose 20 mg/kg 6 hourly (15 mg/kg if < 3 months; 8 hourly if > 36 wks and 12 hourly if < 36 wks gestation) Maximum dose − 80 mg/kg/24 h (60 mg/kg if < 3 months)	Suppositories 60, 125, 250, 500 mg and 1 g	
Ibuprofen 4–10 mg/kg every 6–8 hours	Oral suspension 100 mg/5 ml Tablets 200 mg and 400 mg	Do not use if less than 1 year old
Diclofenac 500 micrograms to 1 mg/kg every 8–12 hours	Tablets 25 mg and 50 mg Suppositories 12·5 mg, 25 mg, 50 mg, 100 mg	CAUTION in asthmatics and patients with renal impairment Contra-indications: SHOCK Bleeding disorders and hypersensitivity to aspirin
Dihydrocodeine 500 micrograms/kg/dose 4–6 hourly	Tablets 30 mg Elixir 10 mg/5 ml	CAUTION with liver impairment and head injuries May lead to constipation. Consider prophylactic lactulose
Codeine phosphate 500 micrograms to 1 mg/kg/dose 4–6 hourly	Tablets 15 mg, 30 mg Elixir 25 mg/5 ml	CODEINE MUST NOT BE GIVEN IV AS IT CAN REDUCE CARDIAC OUTPUT THROUGH HISTAMINE RELEASE

NSAIDs/dihydrocodeine/paracetamol can be used in combination

Oral morphine for severe pain in infants and children

Drug	Preparation
ORAMORPH	
1–12 months 100 micrograms/kg every 4 hours Maximum of 5 doses in 24 hours	Mixture 10 mg/5 ml
1–12 yrs 200–500 micrograms/kg/ dose every 4 hours	Tablets: 10 mg, 20 mg
Over 12 yrs 10–15 mg. every 4 hours	
Single dose prior to painful procedure may be useful	
For long term severe pain, give slow release as the total daily dose of short acting in 2 divided doses (usually 200–500 micrograms/kg every 12 hours)	Slow release tablets: 5 mg, 10 mg, 30 mg, 60 mg, 100 mg Slow release suspension: Sachets 20 mg, 30 mg, 60 mg, 100 mg, 200 mg

Subcutaneous intermittent morphine

Technique	Dose
22/24 gauge subcutaneous cannula Suitable sites: Uppermost arm abdominal skin. Give dose slowly over 5 minutes. Flush with 0·3 ml 0·9% saline (can be sited at the time of surgery)	Morphine: 100–200 micrograms/kg × 3 hourly Maximum 6 × /24 h

Intermittent IV bolus morphine in infants and children

Age	Loading dose	Subsequent doses (GIVE SLOWLY OVER 10 MIN)
1–3 months	100 micrograms/kg over 30 min	25 micrograms/kg/dose × 6 hourly
3–6 months	100 micrograms/kg over 30 min	50 micrograms/kg/dose × 6 hourly
5–12 months	100 micrograms/kg over 30 min	100 micrograms/kg/dose × 6 hourly
1–12 yrs	100–200 micrograms/kg over 5–20 min	100–200 micrograms/kg × 4 hourly
> 12 yrs	2·5 to 10 mg over 5–20 min	2·5–10 mg × 4 hourly

Intravenous infusion of morphine in infants and children

Morphine dose 1 mg/kg made up to 50 mls 0·9% saline.
Then 1 ml/h = 20 micrograms/kg/h, 2 ml/h = 40 micrograms/kg/h,
3 ml/h = 60 micrograms/kg/h, etc.

Loading dose	Technique	Continuous infusion
1–12 months 100 micrograms/kg over 30–60 minutes	Use dedicated cannula	10–40 micrograms/kg/h
> 1 year 100 to 200 micrograms/ kg over 5–20 minutes	**Requires one to one nursing. Monitor the following:** Syringe movement Signs of inflammation at site of infusion Urinary retention	For most situations start at 10 micrograms/kg/ hour and increase in 5 micrograms/kg/h units **Major surgery:** Start at 20 micrograms/kg/h adjust according to pain control

Local Anaesthesia issues

**Maximum doses lidocaine = 3 mg/kg (7 mg/kg with 1 in
200 000 epinephrine)**
**Vasoconstrictors must not be used in tissues with end arteries
for examples: finger, toes, penis**

Toxicity
- Related to dose
- If accidentally administered IV, therefore drawback before
  infusing and ensure needle is not in a vein
- Can be absorbed through mucous membranes in sufficient
  concentrations to be toxic.
- Systemic effects
  neurological: nausea, restless, convulsions,
  cardiovascular: bradycardia, hypotension
- Earliest sign = tingling of lips

Sedative drugs

Drug	Route	Onset	Duration	Dose
Chloral Hydrate Liquid 100 mg/ml Suppositories 100 mg and 500 mg	Oral or Rectal	30 min–1 h	1–2 h	30 mg /kg for night sedation 50–70 mg/kg for procedures 70–100 mg/kg for scans MAXIMUM DOSE 2 g

COMMENTS: Chloral Hydrate is better for younger babies < 18 months or < 15 kg but may paradoxically worsen agitation (e.g. in Down's Syndrome)

Drug	Route	Onset	Duration	Dose
Midazolam Injection 10 mg in 2 ml or 5 ml	Slow injection IV over 5 min	Immediate	30 min to 2 h	100–200 micrograms/kg
	IV infusion Intra-nasal	Immediate 10–30 min	1–2 h	30–300 micrograms/kg/h 200 micrograms/ kg (max.10 mg)
	Sublingual	10–20 min	1–2h	500 micrograms/kg (max.10 mg)

COMMENTS: Benzodiazepines are more suitable for children > 18 mths

Ketamine

Only to be used by those experienced in airway maintenance and full resuscitation

- 1 mg/kg slow IV bolus (over 2–5 minutes)
- Repeat using half dose (500 micrograms/kg) after 15 minutes

- For IM induction use 5–10 mg/kg
- For infusion purposes aim to make up a solution of 1mg/ml (for example 500 mg in 500 ml bag of 5% dextrose or 0·9% saline)
- Adjust to response. Infuse IV at 10–45 micrograms/kg/min

Marked tachyphalaxis can occur with infusions lasting > 30–60 minutes.

Drug infusions in severely ill or injured children

Aminophylline: 5% dextrose or 0·9% saline

Loading dose (do not give if theophylline has been received in the last 24 hours) IV infusion over 20–30 minutes. 5 mg/kg for < 12 years and 250–500 mg in total if > 12 years
Then 1 mg/kg/h if < 12 years and 500 micrograms/kg/h if > 12 years: this is equivalent to 50 mg/kg in 50 ml run at 1 ml/hour for < 12 year and 0·5 ml/hour for > 12 years.

Atracurium: 0·9% saline

500 micrograms/kg initial loading dose then
200 micrograms/kg supplements as required or
200–600 micrograms/kg/h
Maximum concentration 500 micrograms/ml

Diamorphine: 0·9% saline or water; use within 24 hours

Intravenous 10–30 micrograms/kg/h: this is equivalent to 2 mg/kg in 50 ml run at 0·25–0·75 ml/h
Subcutaneous 20-100 micrograms/kg/h: this is equivalent to 2 mg/kg in 50 ml run at 0·5–2·5 ml/h

Dobutamine: 5% dextrose or 0·9% saline. Do not mix with bicarbonate

2–20 micrograms/kg/min: this is equivalent to
30 mg/kg in 50 ml run at 0·2–2 ml/hour (maximum concentration of 5 mg/ml)

Dopamine: 5% dextrose or 0.9% saline or neat (ideally via a central line). Do not mix with bicarbonate.

Can be mixed with dobutamine.

2–20 micrograms/kg/min (renal = up to 5 micrograms/kg/min): this is equivalent to

30 mg/kg in 50 ml run at 0·2–2 ml/h

Epinephrine: 5% dextrose or 0.9% saline. Do not mix with bicarbonate.

0·05–2 micrograms/kg/min: this is equivalent to

0·3 ml/kg of 1:1000 (300 micrograms/kg) in 50-ml run at 0·5–20 ml/h

As short term measure, place 1 mg (1 ml of 1 in 1000 epinephrine) in 50 ml 0·9% saline. Give 2–5 ml (40–100 micrograms) in a child (depending on size) and 1 ml (20 micrograms) to an infant < 1 year. Give IV slowly. Repeat as required (ideally with ECG monitoring).

Fentanyl: 5% dextrose or 0.9% saline or Neat

1–8 micrograms/kg/h: this is equivalent to

200 micrograms/kg in 50 ml at 0·25–2 ml/h

or Neat (50 micrograms/ml): run at 0·02–0·16 ml/kg/h

Ketamine: 5% dextrose or 0.9% saline

10–45 micrograms/kg/min this is equivalent to

50 mg/kg in 50 ml run at 0·6–2·7 ml/h (maximum concentration 50 mg/ml)

Midazolam: 5% dextrose or 0.9% saline or neat

1–6 micrograms/kg/min (60–360 micrograms/kg/h): this is equivalent to 6 mg/kg in 50 ml run at 0·5–3 ml/h

or Neat: (5 mg/ml): run at 0·012–0·072 ml/kg/h

Morphine: 5% dextrose or 0.9% saline

10–60 micrograms/kg/h: this is equivalent to

1 mg/kg in 50 ml run at 0·5–3 ml/h

Nitroprusside: 5% dextrose only **Protect infusion from light. Discard after 24 hours**

0·2–8 micrograms/kg/min: this is equivalent to
3 mg/kg in 50 ml run at 0·2–8 ml/h

Propofol: Neat (*Beware* use in older children > 3 years only). Can be diluted with 5% glucose.

Neat (10 mg/ml): run at 0·2 ml/kg/h (= 2 mg/kg/h) increase as required (maximum 10 mg/kg/h)

Prostacyclin (Epoprostenol): 0·9% saline only. Incompatible with glucose.

5–20 nanograms/kg/min: this is equivalent to
12 micrograms/kg in 50 ml run at 1·25–5 ml/h

Prostaglandin E_2 (Dinoprostone): 5% dextrose or 0·9% saline. Use separate IV line

5–10 fold higher doses of prostaglandin E_2 have been used to re-open the ductus arteriosus but this commonly causes apnoea
5–20 nanograms/kg/min: this is equivalent to
12 micrograms/kg in 50 ml run at 1·25–5 ml/h

Salbutamol: 5% dextrose or 0·9% saline

0·6–5 micrograms/kg/min: this is equivalent to
3 mg/kg in 50 ml run at 0·6–5 ml/h

Thiopental – reconstituted with water to give 25 mg/ml

Can be further diluted with 5% dextrose or 0·9% saline
2–8 mg/kg/h this is equivalent to
25 mg/ml: run at 0·08–0·32 ml/kg/h

Vecuronium: 5% dextrose or 0·9% saline

1–3 micrograms/kg/min: this is equivalent to
3 mg/kg in 50 ml run at 1–3 ml/h

Blood transfusion

Only when essential

Warm pack contact with mother's skin

Do not use blood stored for > 35 days at 2–6 degrees C or out of fridge for > 2 hours or visibly spoiled (plasma must not be pink, redcells not purple or black) or bag open or leaking.

Check correct group and patient's name and numbers and blood group are identical on label and form

Needle/catheter 22 gauge or larger to prevent clotting

If heart failure give 1 mg/kg of frusemide IV at start of transfusion unless hypovolaemic shock is also present.

In severe malnutrition consider partial exchange (see page 89).

Record baseline temperature and pulse rate

Do not allow single unit to go in > 4 hours

Infants or those in heart failure, control flow with in-line burette

Record observations every 30 minutes looking for heart failure and transfusion reactions

Record quantities given

Indications:

- Severe anaemia (Hb < 4 g/dl)
- Impending or overt cardiac failure if Hb < 6 g/dl
- Hyper-parasitaemia in malaria if Hb < 6 g/dl
- In sickle cell disease
  a) if Hb < 5 g/dl or severe infection present
  b) Cerebrovascular accident (CVA) (regardless of Hb)
  c) Priapism (regardless of Hb)
- Children in cardiac failure from severe anaemia (gallop, enlarged liver, raised JVP and fine basal creps from pulmonary oedema)
- Severe chronic haemolytic anaemia such as Thalassaemia Major

• Following acute severe blood loss when 20–30% of the total blood volume of 80 ml/kg is lost and bleeding is continuing – remember Hb can initially be normal

Acute blood loss

Give 10–20 ml/kg of whole blood through wide bore cannula or central venous line.
Estimate infusion rate for continuing transfusion using:-

• an estimate of blood lost
• an estimate of continuing loss
• vital signs

Top-up Transfusion for severe anaemia

WHOLE BLOOD:	20 ml/kg (increases Hb by 25% as blood volume 80 ml/kg) **or** required volume (ml) = weight (kg) × 4 × desired rise in Hb (g/dl)
PACKED RED CELLS:	15 ml/kg or required volume (ml) = weight (kg) × 3 × desired rise in Hb (g/dl)

Blood giving set = 15 drops/ml
Thus mls/hour divided by 4 = drops/min
Use a burette in infants or where too rapid infusion could be dangerous (incipient or actual heart failure).

Commonly available crystalloid fluids

Fluid	Na + (mmol/l)	K + (mmol/l)	Cl − (mmol/l)	Energy (kcal/l)	Comments
Isotonic crystalloid fluids					
Saline 0·9%	150	0	150	0	
Saline 0·18%, dextrose 4%	30	0	30	160	
Dextrose 5%	0	0	0	200	
Hartmann's solution (Ringer's lactate)	131	5	111	0	278 mosm/l Lactate: 29 mmol/l Calcium: 2 mmol/l
Hypertonic crystalloid solutions					
Saline 0·45%, dextrose 5%	75	0	75	200	
Dextrose 10%	0	0	0	400	555 mosm/l

Commonly available colloid fluids

Colloid solutions	Na + (mmol/l)	K + (mmol/l)	Ca ++ (mmol/l)	Duration of action (hours)	Comments
Albumin 4·5%	150	1	0	6	Protein buffers
Gelofusin	154	<1	<1	3	Gelatine
Haemaccel	145	5	12·5	3	Gelatine
Pentastarch	154	0	0	7	Hydroxyethyl starch

Some useful information

1. Percentage solution = grams in 100 ml e.g. 10% dextrose = 10 g in 100 ml
2. 30% NaCl   = 5 mmol/ml each of Na and Cl
   0·9% NaCl   = 0·154 mmol/ml each of Na and Cl
   15% KCl   = 2 mmol/ml strong KCl
   (15 g/100 ml)
   10% Ca Gluconate = 0·225 mmol/ml
   (10 g/100 ml)
   8·4% $NaHCO_3$ = 1 mmol Na and HCO_3/ml
   1 ml/h 0·9% saline = 3·7 mmol Na in 24 hours
3. Serum Osmolality = 2 (Na + K) + glucose + urea
                            (normally 276–295 mosm/l)

FENa (fractional excretion of sodium)

Urinary and plasma **sodium** and **creatinine** concentrations of a spot sample distinguish pre- from established renal failure and diagnose hypovolaemia (check plasma and urine creatinine are in the same units)

FENa (%) = U/P sodium × P/U creatinine × 100

Systolic blood pressures at different ages (mm Hg)

	1 month	1 year	5 years	10 years	15 years
Mean	60	80	90	105	115
Upper limit of normal	80	100	110	120	130
needs urgent treatment	110	130	140	150	160

Normal values for laboratory measurements

Haemoglobin

Age	Hb g/dl
1–3 days	14·5–22·5
2 weeks	14·5–18·0
6 months	10·0–12·5
1–5 years	10·5–13·0
6–12 years	11·5–15·0
12–18 years (male)	13·0–16·0
12–18 years (female)	12·0–16·0

Platelets

Age	Platelets 10^9/litre
Newborn	84–478
Child	150–400

ESR

All ages	0–10 mm/hr

Total WBC

Age	x 10^9/litre
1–2 days	9·0–34·0
Neonates	6·0–19·5
1–3 years	6·0–17.5
4–7 years	5·5–15·5
8–13 years	4·5–13·5

Lymphocytes

>1·year	Median 4·1–6·0 × 10^9

Normal development

Age	Normal achievements in development
Birth	Focuses with eyes and responds to sound
4–6 weeks	Social smile
6–7 months	Sits without support, transfers objects
9–10 months	Gets to sitting position, pulls to stand, pincer grasp, waves good bye
12 months	Stands, walks with one hand held, 2–3 words, stranger anxiety
15 months	Walks, drinks from cup
18 months	Walks upstairs, 10 words, feeds with spoon
2 years	Runs, draws straight line, 2 word sentences
3 years	Draws circle, draws cross, dresses in simple clothes without assistance
4 years	Hops on one leg, draws cross, fluent speech

Warning signs in development

Age	Warning sign
10 weeks	Not smiling
3 months	Not responding to noises or voice, not focusing on face, not vocalising, not lifting up head when lying prone
6 months	Not interested in people, noises, toys, does not laugh or smile, squint, hand preference, primitive reflexes still present
9–12 months	Not sitting, not saying "baba", "mama", not imitating speech sounds, no pincer grasp
18 months	Not walking, no words, still mouthing, no eye contact, not naming familiar objects, not interested in animals, cars and other objects, passive – no moving about exploring, running, climbing, excessive periods of rocking and head banging
3 years	Unaware of surroundings, not imitating adult activities, little or no speech, long periods of repetitive behaviour, unable to follow simple command
4 years	Unintelligible speech
At any age	*Parental concern, regression of acquired skills*

Blood Chemistry

Substance	Age	Value range
Albumin	Pre term	18–30 g/l
	Full term (< 1 week)	25–34 g/l
	<5 years	39–50 g/l
	5–19 years	40–53 g/l
Amylase	All ages	30–100 units per litre
Bicarbonate	All ages	Arterial: 21–28 mmol/l
		Venous: 22–29 mmol/l
Bilirubin conjugated	> 1 year	0–3·4 micromol/l
Calcium		Total Ionised
	0–24 h	2·3–2·65 mmol/l 1·07–1·27 mmol/l
	24 h–4 days	1·75–3·0 mmol/l 1·00–1·17 mmol/l
	4–7 days	2·25–2·73 mmol/l 1·12–1·23 mmol/l
	child	2·15–2·70 mmol/l 1·12–1·23 mmol/l
Chloride	Neonate	97–110 mmol/l
	Child	98–106 mmol/l
Creatinine	Neonate	27–88 micromol/l
	Infant	18–35 micromol/l
	child	27–62 micromol/l

Continued

Continued

Substance	Age	Value range
Glucose	Preterm	1·4–3·3 mmol/l
	0–24 h	2·2–3·3 mmol/l
	Infant	2·8–5·0 mmol/l
	Child	3·3–5·5 mmol/l
Magnesium	0–7 days	0·48–1·05 mmol/l
	7 days–2 years	0·65–1·05 micromol/l
	2–14 years	0·60–0·95 mmol/l
Osmolality	Child	Serum 276–295 mosmol/l
Alkaline phosphatase	< 9 years	145–420 units per litre
Inorganic phosphorus	0–5 days	1·55– 2·65 mmol/l
	1–3 years	1·25–2·10 mmol/l
	4–11 years	1·20–1·80 mmol/l
	12–15 years	0·95–1·75 mmol/l
Potassium	< 2 months	3·0–7·0 mmol/l
	2–12 months	3·6–6·0 mmol/l
	>1 year	3·5–5·0 mmol/l

Substance	Age	Valu range
Sodium	Newborn	134–146 mmol/l
	Infant	139–146 mmol/l
	Child	138–146 mmol/l
Retinol/vitamin A	1–6 years	0.70 – 1.5 micromol/l
	7–12 years	0.9 – 1.7 micromol/l
	13–19 years	0.9 – 2.5 micromol/l
Urea	Child	2.5–6.6 mmol/l
Zinc	Child	9.8–18.1 micromol/l

Paediatric electrocardiography

Heat rate and rhythm

Atrial hypertrophy P wave in lead II > 0.28 mV

PR interval, > 0.12 seconds infancy and > 0.16 seconds in childhood = prolonged

Mean frontal QRS axis : Superior axis = QRS forces in AVF negative

: Mean 135° day 1, 110° neonatal, 65° child

RVH:	Positive T wave in V_4R, V_1V_2 from 7 days of life until puberty	
LVH:	Inverted T waves V_4, V_5, V_6	
RVH:	R waves in V_4R	> 15 mV < 3 months of age
		> 10 mV > 3 months
LVH:	R waves in V_6	> 20 mV < 3 months
		> 25 mV > 3 months
3 patterns:	neonatal	= R > S in V_4R, V_1
		= S > R in V_5, V_6
	Infant	= R > S in V_4R or V_1 and V_6
	Adult	= R < S in V_4R or V_1
		= S > R in V_6
Biventricular hypertrophy		= R + S in V4 = >70 mV

Index

Abbreviations; ICP, intracranial pressure.

ABC(DE) *see* airway;
        breathing; circulation;
        disability; exposure; life
        support
abdomen, acute 136–8
accessory respiratory muscle
        use 17
Adelaide Coma Scale 29
adrenal crisis 108–9
adrenaline *see* epinephrine
airway
        assessment and
                management 16,
                151–7
        allergic/anaphylactic
                reactions 35
        intubation *see*
                endotracheal
                intubation
        in life support 9, 11–12
        primary assessment 16
        procedures/equipment
                151–7
        trauma cases 138–9
        in triage 7
        unconscious child 27
        emergency surgical 154–6
        obstruction, signs 139
        upper, problems 68–9
        see also respiratory
                disorders
albendazole 126

alcohol poisoning 42
allergic reactions 35–6
aminophylline 5, 180
amputation, traumatic
        143–4
anaemia
        blood transfusion 88–9,
                184
        iron–deficiency 88–9
analgesia *see* pain relief
anaphylactic shock 35–6
anthelmintics 90, 126
antibiotics
        endocarditis prophylaxis
                71, 72
        intestinal obstruction 138
        malnourished child 84
        meningitis 61, 98–9, 101,
                102–3
        meningococcal disease
                112, 113
        neonatal infections 60,
                61, 99
        tetanus 114
        typhoid 116
anticonvulsants 63
        status epilepticus 37, 38
antidepressant poisoning 43
antimalarials 122–4
antitoxin
        diphtheria 111–12
        venoms 129–30, 131, 132
apnoea, neonatal 58
appendicitis 136
arrhythmias 14–15

defibrillation 168–9
  shock secondary to 25
asthma, acute 69–70
asystole 14
atracurium 180
atropine 44
AVPU response 6, 20–1
  diabetic ketoacidosis 105
  unconscious child 27

benzodiazepine poisoning 42
bicarbonate see sodium
  bicarbonate
bleach ingestion 43
blood cell values 188
blood chemistry 191–3
blood loss see haemorrhage
blood pressure, systolic 7, 187
  assessment 19
  in shock 23
blood transfusion 183–4
  in anaemia 88–9, 184
  exchange 165–7
  in malaria 124
bowel see intestine
brachial vein cannulation 163
brain (incl. cerebrum)
  malaria 122
  oedema 107–8
  supratentorial mass 34
  see also encephalopathy
breastmilk, orogastric 49
breathing (assessment and
    management) 16–18,
    156–8
  allergic/anaphylactic
    reactions 35–6
  efficacy/effectiveness
    18, 57

effort/work of breathing
    17–18, 57
intubation see
    endotracheal
    intubation
  in life support 9, 11
  neonatal 9, 57
  primary assessment 16–18
  procedures/equipment
    156–8
  trauma cases 140
  in triage 7
  unconscious child 27
  see also respiration
burns 145–8
  corrosive chemical 40

caloric response 28
cannulation see vascular
    access
capillary refill 19
  in shock 23
carbamazepine, neonatal 63
carbon monoxide
    poisoning 45
cardiovascular system see
    circulation; heart
catheterisation see
    vascular access
cerebral disorders see brain
cerebrospinal fluid analysis
    (lumbar puncture)
    60–1, 98, 99, 100
cervical spine, trauma cases
    138–9, 139
chest compression 12
  neonatal 9
chest drains 157–8
  empyema 159

chloral hydrate 179
chloride, requirements/
    body fluid contents 5
chlormethiazole 38
circulation
    assessment and
        management 19–20,
        159–69
    in allergic/anaphylactic
        reactions 36
    in dehydration 3–5
    primary assessment
        19–20
    procedures/equipment
        159–69
    in shock 22–3
    in trauma 140–1
    in triage 8
    in unconscious child 27
    collapse, management 85
    inadequacy, effects on
        other organs
        19–20, 23
    raised ICP effects on 21
clonazepam, neonatal 63
codeine phosphate 175
cold water on burns 145
colloid fluids 185
coma 26
    scales 28
convulsions see seizures
cooling, urgent 134
corrosive chemicals 40, 43
cranial nerve assessment 28
cricothyroidotomy 154–6
croup 67, 68
crystalloid fluids 185
cut down, venous 162–3
cyanotic heart disease 73–4

defibrillation 168–9
dehydration 3–4
    in diabetic
        ketoacidosis 105
    septic shock v 83
    in severe malnutrition
        80–3
    treatment see fluid
        management
dengue haemorrhagic
    disease 112
development
    normal 189
    warning signs 190
dexamethasone, raised ICP
    31, 33
dextrose see glucose
diabetic ketoacidosis 104–8
dialysis 96
diamorphine 180
diarrhoea 90–1
diazepam 5
    status epilepticus 38
    tetanus 114
diclofenac 175
diet see nutritional support
dinoprostone 182
diphtheria 111–12
disability (neurological)
    assessment 6, 20–1
    diabetic ketoacidosis 105
    primary assessment
        20–1
    trauma 141
    triage 8
    unconscious child 27
    see also mental status;
        unconscious child
dobutamine 180

dopamine 181
dressings, burns 148
drugs 174–82
    essential 5–6, 180–2
        doses 5–6
        neonatal life support 10
        paediatric life
            support 13
        overdose/poisoning 41–3
    *see also specific (types of)
        drugs*

ECG *see* electrocardiography
electrocardiography
        (ECG) 194
    life support 13
electrolytes
    body fluid contents 5
    disturbances (and their
        correction)
        in gastroenteritis 77–8
        in malnutrition 83
        in renal failure 96
    requirements 5, 49–50
empyema, drainage 159
encephalopathy
    hepatic 93–5
    neonatal hypoxic
        ischaemic 64
endocarditis prophylaxis
        71, 72
endocrine disorders 104–10
endotracheal intubation
        (incl. orotracheal
        11–12, 151–3
    dimensions 3, 11–12, 151
    trauma 139
energy requirements 5
enterocolitis, necrotising 61

envenoming 127–32
environmental emergencies
        126–35
epiglottitis, acute 68
epilepsy, continuous (status
        epilepticus) 37–8
epinephrine (adrenaline) 5
    allergic/anaphylactic
        reactions 36
    asthma 69
    life support 13, 14, 15
        neonates 10
    severe illness or
        trauma 181
epoprostenol 182
erythrocytes (red cells)
        packed 184
    sedimentation rate 188
exchange transfusion 165–7
expiratory noises 17
exposure, trauma 141
eye movements/responses
        (unconscious child) 28
    in coma scales 29

F–75 92
feeding *see* nutritional
support
femoral artery cannulation
        160
fentanyl 181
first aid
    burns 145
    snakebite 127–8
fish, venomous 132
fluid management (incl.
        rehydration) 20–1, 185
    asystole 14
    burns 147–8

commonly available
    fluids 185
dehydration 4
    in gastroenteritis 76–7,
        78–9
    in severe malnutrition
        80–3
    diabetic ketoacidosis
        105–6
    meningitis 99
    pulseless electrical
        activity 14
    renal failure 95, 96
    shock 23–5
    trauma 141
    see also water
fluid requirements 4,
    5, 49

gastroenteritis 75–9
gastrointestinal disorders
    75–92, 90–1, 136–8
    helminths 90, 125
    neonatal 61
Glasgow Coma Scale 29
glucose
    administration (incl.
        dextrose)
        diabetic ketoacidosis
            107
        hyperkalaemia 97
        hypoglycaemia 52,
            53, 86, 109, 124
        meningitis 101
        neonates 52, 53
        blood 192
        low see hypoglycaemia
great arteries, transposition
    74

grunting 17
gunshot wound 144–5

haemoglobin concentrations
    188
haemolytic disease, neonatal
    54
haemorrhage/blood loss
    transfusion 184
    trauma case 140
haemorrhagic disease,
    dengue 112
heart
    asystole 14
    disease/disorders
        circulatory inadequacy
            due to 20
        congenital 57, 73–4
    failure 70–4, 86–7
    massage see chest
        compression
    output, establishing 12
    rate
        normal 7
        in respiratory failure 18
        in shock 22
        see also arrhythmias
helminths 125–6
    intestinal 90, 125
hepatic failure,
    acute 93–5
HIV–related disorders 117
hydrocortisone, adrenal
    crisis 108, 109
hyperkalaemia 96–7
hypernatraemia 77–8
hyperthermia 134
hypoglycaemia 109
    malaria 124

malnourished child 86
neonatal 51–3
hypokalaemia 109–10
diabetic ketoacidosis 104
gastroenteritis 78
hyponatraemia 78
hypopituitarism 108
hypothermia
infants 134–5
malnourished child 85
hypoxic ischaemic
encephalopathy,
neonatal 64

immunisation, rabies
119–21
immunoglobulin
rabies 120
tetanus 114
infants *see also* neonates
hypothermia 134–5
raised intracranial
pressure relief 34
infections (incl. sepsis)
59–61, 111–26
malnourished child 84
meningeal 60–1, 98–102
neonatal 54, 59–61
respiratory 67–8
unconscious/comatose
child 26
screening for 30
see also septic shock
injury *see* trauma
inspiratory noises 17
insulin
diabetic ketoacidosis
106–7
meningitis 97

intestine 61, 136–8
parasites 90, 125
intracranial pressure (ICP),
raised 27, 32–4
effects/presentation 21,
32–3
management 31,
33–4, 34
intraosseous needle 166–7
intravenous access
see venous access
intubation *see* endotracheal
intubation
intussusception 136–7
iodide supplements 88
ipecac 40–1
iron
deficiency 88–9
poisoning 41–2

jaundice, neonatal 54–6
jellyfish stings 132
jugular vein cannulation
external 159
internal 161–2

kerosene ingestion 44
ketamine 179–80, 181
ketoacidosis, diabetic 104–8
kidney failure, acute 95–7
kwashiorkor, dermatosis
of 90

laboratory tests and values
188–93
neonatal infections 59
normal values 188
lactose intolerance 90
laryngoscope 151, 152

lead poisoning 45
lidocaine 178
life support (incl. ABC of
    resuscitation) 11–13
  neonatal 9–10
    drugs 10
  see also specific conditions
listeriosis, headaches 98
liver failure, acute 93–5
local anaesthetics 178
lorazepam 38
lumbar puncture,
    60–1, 98, 99, 100
lymphocyte count 188

malaria 91, 121–5
  cerebral 122
malnutrition 79–92
mannitol 6, 31, 33, 107, 108
measles 88, 88–9, 116–19
mebendazole 90, 126
meningitis 60–1, 98–102
meningococcal disease 112
mental status
  in circulatory
      inadequacy 20
  in respiratory failure 18
  see also disability
      assessment;
      unconscious child
metabolic disorders 104–10
  coma 26
  neonatal seizures 62
micronutrient deficiencies 88
midazolam 179
  severe illness/trauma 181
  status epilepticus 38
mid upper arm
    circumference 173

missile wounds 144–5
morphine 6, 174–8, 181
motor function/response
    (unconscious child) 28
  in coma scales 29

naloxone 174
nasogastric feeding 80
near drowning 132–4
necrotising enterocolitis 61
needle cricothyroidotomy
    154–5
needle pericardiocentesis
    167
needle thoracentesis 156–7
neonates 47–64
  life support *see* life support
  meningitis 60–1, 99
neurological assessment *see*
    disability assessment
neurological infections *see*
    malaria; meningitis
nitroprusside 182
nutritional disorders 79–92
nutritional support
    (feeding/diet)
  malnutrition 80, 82, 91–2
  meningitis 101
  neonatal respiratory
distress 58
  renal failure 96

ocular movements *see* eye
    movements
oculocephalic reflex 28
oculovestibular
    response 28
oedema, cerebral 107–8
opiate/opioids 174–8

overdose 39
organophosphorus
    poisoning 44
osmotic diarrhoea 91
oxygen, allergic/anaphylactic
    reactions 36

pain relief 174–6
    tetanus 115
paracetamol 175
    poisoning 42, 95
paraldehyde
    neonatal 63
    status epilepticus 38
parasites *see* helminths;
    malaria
pericardiocentesis,
    needle 167
petroleum compounds,
    ingestion 44
phenobarbitone
    neonatal 63
    status epilepticus 38
phenytoin
    neonatal 63
    status epilepticus 38
phototherapy 55, 56
pituitary hypofunction 108
platelet counts 188
pleural empyema,
    drainage 159
pleural tap 158–9
pneumococcus
    (*S. pneumoniae*) 98, 99
poisoning (toxicology)
    39–45
    paracetamol 42, 95
    unconscious child 30
    see also envenoming

potassium
    administration 109–10
        in diabetic ketoacidosis
            106
    body fluid contents 5
    in colloid/crystalloid
        fluids 185
    requirements 5, 50
    see also hyperkalaemia;
        hypokalaemia
pralidoxime 44
propofol 182
prostacyclin 182
prostaglandin E2 182
protein requirements 5
pulmonary blood flow,
    low 74
pulseless electrical
    activity 14–15
pulseless ventricular
    tachycardia 15
pulse volume 19
    in shock 23
pupillary reactions 21
    unconscious child 28

quinine 123

rabies 119–21
recession (chest) 17
red cells *see* erythrocytes
renal failure, acute 95–7
ReSoMal 81, 82
respiration
    raised ICP effects 21
    trauma cases 140
    unconscious child 28–30
    see also breathing
respiratory disorders 67–70

neonatal 57–8
respiratory distress, neonatal, causes 57
respiratory failure, physiological effects 18
respiratory rate
   abnormal 17
   normal 7
resuscitation *see* airway; breathing; circulation; disability; exposure; life support
rewarming *see* warming
rheumatic fever, acute 71

Safe approach 11
salbutamol 6, 70, 182
salicylate poisoning 42–3
saphenous vein cannulation 163
scorpion stings 130–1
sedation 179
seizures/convulsions
   hypoglycaemic child 86
   meningitis 101
   neonatal 62–3
   repeated (status epilepticus) 37–8
septic shock 84
   severe dehydration *v* 83
   see also infections
shock 22–5
   anaphylactic 35–6
   malaria 124–5
   septic *see* septic shock
skin
   colour
      in circulatory inadequacy 19

in respiratory failure 18
   kwashiorkor 90
snakebite 127–30
sodium
   body fluid contents 5
   in colloid/crystalloid fluids 185
   fractional excretion 186
   requirements 5, 49
   supplements 49
   see also hypernatraemia; hyponatraemia
sodium bicarbonate 6
   in diabetic ketoacidosis 106
   in hyperkalaemia 97
   in life support 13, 14, 15
sodium valproate, neonatal 63
spasms, tetanus 114
spider bites 131–2
spinal cord injury 143
spine, cervical, trauma cases 138–9, 139
status epilepticus 37–8
steroids
   adrenal crisis 108, 109
   raised ICP 31, 33
Streptococcus pneumoniae (pneumococcus) 98, 99
subclavian vein cannulation 162
supraventricular tachycardia, shock secondary to 25
surface area, body, estimation 173
systolic blood pressure *see* blood pressure

tachycardia/tachyarrhythmia
    shock secondary to 25
    ventricular *see* ventricular
        tachycardia
tetanus 114–15
thiopental 182
thiopentone 38
thoracentesis, needle 156–7
toxicology *see* antitoxin;
    poisoning
tracheal intubation *see*
    endotracheal intubation
transposition of great
    arteries 74
trauma/injury 138–48
    drug infusions 180–2
triage 7–8
tricyclic antidepressant
    poisoning 43
tuberculosis (TB) 91
    meningeal 98–9
turpentine ingestion 44
typhoid fever 115–16

umbilical vein catheterisation
    164–5
unconscious child 26–34
    hypoglycaemia 86
    see also disability
        assessment; mental
        status
UNCRC standards xi
urinary output in circulatory
    inadequacy 20, 23

vaccine, rabies 119–20, 121
vascular access 159–65

intraosseous 166–7
    in life support 13
vecuronium 182
venoms 127–32
venous access 159, 161–5
    in life support 13
ventilation 12
    see also breathing
ventricular tachycardia
    pulseless 15
    shock secondary to 25
verbal response in coma
    scales 29
vital signs, normal values 7
vitamin deficiency and
    supplementation 88–9
vomiting, induced 40–1

warming/rewarming 134–5
    near drowning 133–4
water (fluid) requirements
    4, 5, 49
    see also fluid requirements
weight 3
    body surface area and 173
    for length and height
        171–2
white cell count
    blood 188
    CSF 100
worms *see* helminths

xerophthalmia 88–9, 119

zinc supplements 88